I.K. STEELE is a professor in the Department of History at the University of Western Ontario.

The letters of Joseph Cruttenden, London merchant-apothecary, form a unique document in early modern economic, medical, and social history. Cruttenden, who carried on trade in colonial America and the British West Indies, did not represent the powerful merchant houses that handled much of the colonial trade as commission agents and staple traders. He was one of the thousands of small traders whose names survive, like rows of miniature tombstones, only in the English portbooks.

The remedies his colonial customers ordered suggest that these physicians, clerics, and merchant apothecaries were better informed about new drugs and practices than has been assumed. Cruttenden's letters provide a rare opportunity to evaluate the pharmacy of his time, in terms not of huge pharmacopoeias but of the ingredients and remedies actually sought by practitioners. Though almost all his drugs, elixirs, and cordials have since been discarded as worthless, if not harmful, he received few complaints about their failure to perform the feats claimed in the pharmacopoeias, and he invariably made a vigorous defence of the 'goodness' of what he had sent.

Cruttenden's business practices required more frequent defence in fact than his medicines, and as result the letters provide a detailed picture of the small trader's methods and objectives. Although he specialized in drugs and medicine, he sent many other goods and received a variety of colonial products in return. He offered his customers several methods of payment and discussed insurance, the state of the market for colonial commodities, and smuggling practices.

In frank and engaging style, Cruttenden reveals a little about himself, a great deal about the drug and medicine trade, and even more about the business practices of a small trader in England's Atlantic empire.

EDITED BY I.K. STEELE

Atlantic Merchant-Apothecary

LETTERS OF JOSEPH CRUTTENDEN
1710-1717

UNIVERSITY OF TORONTO PRESS
TORONTO AND BUFFALO

© University of Toronto Press 1977
Toronto and Buffalo
Printed in Canada

Library of Congress Cataloging in Publication Data

Cruttenden, Joseph.
  Atlantic merchant-apothecary.

  Includes bibliographical references and index.
  1. Cruttenden, Joseph. 2. Pharmacists – England
  – London – Correspondence. 3. Drug trade – England –
  History. I. Steele, Ian Kenneth. II. Title.
  RS73.C7A4 1977   382'.45'615094212   77-2832
  ISBN 0-8020-5364-5

This book has been published during the
Sesquicentennial year of the University of Toronto

In memory of Jack Lees,
curiosity and wisdom, without his share of time

Contents

Acknowledgements

Joseph Cruttenden himself has offered an uncommon opportunity to see the concerns of a small London trader in England's Atlantic empire. Richard Rawlinson (1690-1755) gave a place in his mammoth collection to the small, leatherbound 'Letterbook of J.C.' and bequeathed it to the safety and care of the Bodleian Library.

For helping to unravel the identity of 'J.C.,' surely the most common monogram in Christendom, I am particularly grateful to Dr A.E.J. Hollaender of Guildhall Library. Mr Ian Baxter of India Office Records, Dr John Blake of the National Library of Medicine, Bethesda, Maryland, and my colleague Dr C.W. Gowdey were all generous with their special knowledge. Of those who helped in preparing the text and notes, I am particularly indebted to Terence Wister and Mrs G.B. McCall, as well as Margaret Parker of University of Toronto Press. Bodleian Library kindly permitted publication of their manuscript, and both the Canada Council and the University of Western Ontario sponsored research. The book has been published with the assistance of grants from the university's J.B. Smallman Memorial Fund for Publication in the Humanities and Social Sciences and from the Humanities Research Council of Canada, using funds provided by the Canada Council, and grants to the University of Toronto Press from the Andrew W. Mellon Foundation and the University of Toronto. Cruttenden and I share responsibility for what follows; the letters are his and the errors are mine.

I.K.S.
University of Western Ontario

Abbreviations

Bull. of Hist. of Med. – *Bulletin of the History of Medicine*
CSPC – *Calendar of State Papers, Colonial Series*
DNB – *Dictionary of National Biography*
EHR – *English Historical Review*
Ency. Brit. – *Encyclopedia Britannica*, 11th ed., 29 vols. (New York, 1910-11)
GL – Guildhall Library, London, England
J. Hist. of Med. – *Journal of the History of Medicine and Allied Sciences*
J. Econ. Hist. – *Journal of Economic History*
OED – *Oxford English Dictionary*
Statutes – Danby Pickering, *The Statutes at Large from Magna Carta to 1806*, 46
    vols. (Cambridge 1762-1807)
TRHS – *Transactions* of the Royal Historical Society

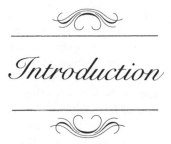

Introduction

Joseph Cruttenden's letterbook is a unique and many-faceted document in social, medical, and economic history. Cruttenden seems to have been a small trader of limited education, who founded no dynasty and wielded no political power in England or in the colonies. Indeed, he was obscure enough that for two hundred years after his death he has been identified only as 'JC', the initials with which he closed copies of his letters. Cruttenden does not represent those powerful merchant houses that handled much of the colonial trade as commission agents and staple traders. He is rather one of the thousands of traders whose names survive, like rows of miniature tombstones, only in the English portbooks. His letters reveal a little about himself, a good deal about the drug and medicine trade to the English colonies, which was his specialty, and even more about the business practices of a small trader in England's Atlantic empire.

Born (c. 1660?) the son of Joseph Cruttenden, gent., of Cranbrook, Kent,[1] young Joseph was apprenticed to the mercantile craft of apothecary, as were many gentlemen's sons.[2] He served a seven-year apprenticeship near home, perhaps under Thomas Cruttenden, apothecary, of the same place.[3] By October 1684 he had moved to London and was bound to an apothecary, Benjamin Bouchier (or Bourchier),[4] for eight more years. But Cruttenden applied for the freedom of the London Society of Apothecaries, was examined, approved, and made free by redemption on 4 January 1686/7.[5]

---

1 GL MS 8200/3, 145
2 See D.V. Glass 'Socio-economic Status and Occupations in the City of London at the end of the Seventeenth Century' in *Studies in London History* ed. A.E.J. Hollaender and William Kellaway (London 1969) 388n.
3 GL, MS 8200/4, 142
4 GL, MS 8200/3, 145
5 GL, MS 8203/3, 217, 222

From his surviving letters it seems clear that he became more of a 'druggist' than an 'apothecary' in the terms of his time. 'A Druggist,' remarked *The London Tradesman*, 'is not supposed to know anything of the Uses or Properties of Drugs: He only buys them as a Merchant, and disposes of them as a Commodity.'[6] Druggists did, in fact, prepare medical compounds for sale, and Cruttenden repeatedly indicates that this was the more profitable, but less common, feature of his business.[7] Although he might have kept specialized copybooks, the colonial emphasis of his overseas trade is supported by his title page, which read simply 'Coppys of Letters 1709/10.' He had some English wholesale drug trade,[8] but his focus upon selling drugs to the English plantations may have started as early as the mid-1690s.[9] Fifteen years later he assured a new colonial customer, 'my busynesse lyes much wholesale beyond sea'[10] while castigating a tardy customer with 'I hope I shall learne att last to bee wiser then trust my effects abroad where I allways meet with disapoyntments.'[11]

What sort of a man, and historical witness, was Joseph Cruttenden? By his own characterization he was candid, fair, concerned about his family, and without pretensions except pride in his work. Although his is the only evidence left on numerous issues, the letterbook certainly puts him in a clearer and less flattering light than an autobiographical memoir might have done.[12] His religious views cannot be determined; his declining to wear a wig is at best a vague clue.[13] His most sustained reference to God was his warning to an errant Jamaican debtor: 'I would have you remember that tho you are att a great distance from me and soe may thinke yourself secure yet the eye of God is upon you and you must give an account to him.'[14] Both ethics and business sense mattered enough to provoke very frank comments from Cruttenden. From what can be verified about his own statements, Cruttenden might have exaggerated but he did not lie. His long, losing battle to maintain prices without losing customers suggests a merchant in stiff competition, and

---

6 R. Campbell *The London Tradesman* (London 1747) 62-3
7 See below, letters 88 and 111 concerning preparing compounds.
8 See below, letters 29, 31, and 81.
9 See below, letters 47 and 81. He imported quantities of ginger and sugar from Barbados in 1696 (Public Record Office, London, E 190/158/1, 396).
10 See below, letter 63.
11 See below, letter 45.
12 See J.D. Marshall's excellent edition of *The Autobiography of William Stout of Lancaster, 1665-1752* (Manchester 1967).
13 See below, letter 4.
14 See below, letter 57.

one who was too dispensable to indulge in sharp practices even if he had wanted to. His abilities were adequate for his calling,[15] but his knowledge of contemporary drugs and medicines was not outstanding.[16] Cruttenden's mathematics was usually sufficient, though he sent one customer a free hat which the latter had claimed because Cruttenden made a mistake in accounting at his own expense. Cruttenden wrote an engaging business letter, and could usually trade Latin phrases with such of his customers as chose to display their learning. Although he shared the human weaknesses of exaggeration and error, his testimony seems generally reliable.

Prosperity would have been an interesting test of Cruttenden's ability and honesty, especially since he so often insisted that his profits were inadequate. This was no period in which to make a fortune in the colonial trades, and many traders lost the struggle for survival or increased their involvement in internal English trade.[17] The eight years of trading recorded in the letterbook were plucked from the midst of a long career. Cruttenden was about fifty in 1710, a married man, apparently with children, and his health may not have been good.[18] Neither wealth nor bankruptcy had moved him by 1727, when he was still living on Newgate Street,[19] and presumably still receiving his mail at the Green Dragon Inn.[20] It was not until 1730/1 that he was named master of his guild,[21] perhaps because the septuagenarian had been more druggist than apothecary. Because his will was apparently destroyed in the burning of Christchurch Newgate in 1940, Cruttenden escapes careful financial assessment, as he escaped fame or notoriety. Whether or not he withdrew from overseas trade, as he repeatedly threatened,[22] wealth escaped him, too.

15 Campbell remarked, 'A Druggist as a mere Seller of Medicines requires no great Head-Piece' (*The London Tradesman* 63).

16 He did not know of Blagrave's eyewater or *unguentum decameron Mindereri*; see letters 95 and 122 respectively.

17 See Richard Grassby 'English Merchant Capitalism in the Late Seventeenth Century: The Composition of Business Fortunes' *Past and Present* 46 (February 1970): 87-107; his 'The Rate of Profit in Seventeenth-Century England' EHR 84 (1969): 721-51; Thomas Hutchinson *The History of the Province of Massachusetts Bay* 2 vols. (Boston 1764-7) 2: 444; Marshall *Autobiography of William Stout* 172.

18 See below, letters 110, 4 and 108 respectively.

19 See the London Livery Poll Book of 1727. I am grateful to Dr Hollaender for this information.

20 Green Dragon inns abounded in Restoration London, but no specific reference to this one has been found. It was almost certainly located in Green Dragon Court, which was north off the lower end of Newgate Street, and just north of St Paul's. It is possible that John Josselyn's *New England's Rarities discovered* printed for G. Widdowes at the Green Dragon in St Paul's Churchyard (London 1672) was printed at the same inn, but at least one other inn could claim that address.

21 GL, MS 8200/5, n.p.

22 See below, letters 45 and 111.

Medical practice in the English empire during the seventeenth and early eighteenth centuries has been difficult to reconstruct, and efforts to do so have been confined primarily to the American continental colonies, especially New England.[23] Medicine there has been regarded as reaching a nadir in this period. Since the learned men of the early migrations were dead by the end of the seventeenth century, the provincial town of Boston had its medical needs served by clerics with some knowledge of physic and by merchant-apothecaries. The arrival of William Douglass, MD, in Boston in 1718 has, with his help, been regarded as the beginning of a new trend. Fully trained European, especially Scottish, doctors would then begin to serve a town just becoming large and sophisticated enough to support some, though not all, of the arriving physicians.[24] Cruttenden's letters to Massachusetts were to merchant apothecaries, clerics, and self-styled physicians, but his trade there does not suggest that these practitioners were ignorant of their craft.

Serving the Massachusetts medical elite, and providing a substantial part of the drugs for Boston,[25] Cruttenden's trade might be said to reflect the best of New England's medical knowledge. His letters, though lacking invoices that would give fuller information, indicate more clearly than do the pharmacopoeias the kind of drugs most imported. Of course, locally grown drugs leave no trace here, except when seeds were ordered from England. Cruttenden's customers were not a representative sample, certainly missing those like Dr Bullivant, Boston apothecary, who 'to the Poor ... always prescribes

23 Provincial English medical practice, the appropriate context, can be seen through: John H. Roach 'Five Early Seventeenth Century English Country Physicians' *J. Hist. of Med.* 20 (1965): 213-25; R.S. Roberts 'The Personnel and Practice of Medicine in Tudor and Stuart England: Part 1, The Provinces' *Medical History* 6 (1962): 363-82; the *Journal of James Yonge, Plymouth Surgeon* ed. F.N.L. Poynter (Hamsden, Conn. 1963); and Claver Morris *The Diary of a West Country Physician* ed. Edmund Hobhouse (London 1934). For American colonial medicine circa 1700 see: Otho T. Beall and R.H. Shryock *Cotton Mather, First Significant Figure in American Medicine* (Baltimore 1954); Michael Kraus 'American and European Medicine in the Eighteenth Century' *Bull. Hist. of Med.* 8 (1940): 679-95; Genevieve Miller 'European Influences in Colonial Medicine' *Ciba Symposia* 8 (1946-7): 511-21; and Whitfield J. Bell Jr. 'Medical Practice in Colonial America' *Bull. Hist. of Med.* 31 (1957): 442-53. New England medicine at that time is studied by Henry Viets *A Brief History of Medicine in Massachusetts* (Boston 1930); John B. Blake *Public Health in the Town of Boston, 1630-1822* (Cambridge, Mass. 1959), and Malcolm S. Beinfield 'The Early New England Doctor: An Adaptation to a Provincial Environment' *Yale Journal of Biology and Medicine* 15 (1942-3): 99 132.
24 See Bell 'Medical Practice in Colonial America' 444, 447; Miller 'European Influences in Colonial Medicine' 511.
25 Henry R. Viets claims that there were fourteen apothecary shops and ten physicians in Boston in 1721, *Brief History* 55, 56. At least three apothecaries were major customers of Cruttenden, without including William Little, George Stewart, or Thomas Greaves in Charlestown.

cheap, but wholesome Medicines, not curing them of a Consumption in ther Bodies, and sending it into their Purses; nor directing them to the East-Indies to look for Drugs, when they may have far better out of their Gardens.'[26] Those who traded with Cruttenden joined in the world trade in drugs, including many drastic and worthless substances, and mixed these drugs themselves. They probably cared for people who could afford to be dissatisfied with, or to supplement, common garden herbs. Yet simples, elixirs, and cordials were the major part of Cruttenden's trade, with chemical therapeutics playing a minor role. These practitioners represented no absolute decline from the medicine of their forebears, though they were as far from the leadership of English medicine as were most provincial English practitioners.[27]

There is some evidence to support the notion that colonial medical usage was out of date in this period. The Rev. John Clayton, ridiculing Virginian doctors in a letter to the Royal Society in 1688, gave a satirical sketch of colonial treatment for flux, ending in the death of the patient.[28] The drugs prescribed in this parody were all a regular part of Cruttenden's colonial trade a quarter of a century later. Cruttenden's own remarks on colonial interest in oil of goldenrod and turpeth[29] suggest that colonial practice was *passé*. Quinine-bearing cinchona bark from Spanish America received its first belated printed endorsement by an English physician by 1672, but was not used in England's American colonies until more than twenty years later.[30] A colonial order for William Salmon's compendious *Synopsis Medicinae* sixteen years after its last printing[31] was but another indication of the difficulties colonial practitioners had in keeping abreast of newer ideas.

Pharmacopoeias were a major reason why the self-taught in England or the colonies could function as apothecaries, and a major determinant of what drugs they could know and use. Nicholas Culpeper's *Pharmacopoeia Londinensis* was an unauthorized translation of the Latin work, adding astrological botany and roundhead sentiments to the legacy of herbals to become an immensely popular book.[32] A shortened version was printed in Boston in 1708,

26 John Dunton *Letters Written from New England* (Boston 1867) 96
27 See Roach 'English Country Physicians' and Roberts 'Medicine in Tudor and Stuart England' in this connection.
28 Reprinted in Peter Force *Tracts and Other Papers* ... 4 vols. (Washington 1836-47) 3, no. 12
29 See below, letters 75 and 79.
30 Miller 'European Influences in Colonial Medicine' 516; W.B. Blanton *Medicine in Virginia in the Seventeenth Century* (Richmond, Va. 1930) 113
31 See below, letters 95 and 101. The fourth, and apparently last, edition of this was in 1699 (DNB 'William Salmon').
32 David L. Cowen 'The Boston Editions of Nicholas Culpeper' *J. Hist. of Med.* 11 (1956): 156-65; Bell 'Medical Practice' 447

becoming the first medical book produced in English America, and a full edition was published there in 1720. This and his *English Physician Enlarged* were common manuals of medicine in the English empire. An inventory of a Boston bookseller in 1700 shows that he stocked Culpeper but had more copies of work by William Salmon (1644-1713), a London empiric who had travelled to New England.[33] Salmon produced his translation of the London Pharmacopoeia in 1678, and it went through several editions between then and 1717.[34] He removed many of Culpeper's additions and, whether or not it was as popular as Culpeper's, Salmon's work is the best single reference for identifying drugs ordered from Cruttenden.

Surprisingly enough, some colonial practitioners were very aware of various new developments. Gamboge was a new oriental drug, first introduced into the 1724 edition of the London Pharmacopoeia, yet colonial practitioners were ordering it from Jamaica in 1710 and Massachusetts in 1713.[35] Stoughton's elixir was being ordered a year before it was patented in England and long before advertisements appeared in Massachusetts papers.[36] Colonial orders for Blagrave's eye water[37] and *Unguentum decameron mindereri*[38] baffled Cruttenden. While this reflects upon his knowledge, it also suggests that colonial apothecaries and physicians learned from correspondents, from ship surgeons, and from emigrating English practitioners and customers. The colonial panacea, Virginia or Seneca snakeroot, destined to become famous in England in the 1730s, was already in use in Boston, but Cruttenden was, quite naturally, unwilling to accept it as a commodity in 1715.[39]

Although almost all of the drugs and medicines of Cruttenden's time have since been discarded as worthless, if not harmful, he received very few complaints about the failure of ingredients to perform the feats claimed for them in the pharmacopoeias. When he was challenged on the quality of his goods, he certainly defended himself vigorously.[40] If the sick were not always cured by the combined power of prayer, placebo, herbal medicine, and the healing power of the body, it was not customary for the clerics and physicians to blame the druggist.

33 See inventory of Michael Perry in *Publications of the Prince Society* 4 (Boston 1867): 314-19, and DNB 'William Salmon.'
34 *Pharmacopoeia Londinensis, or the New London Dispensatory*
35 See below, letter 18 and note 1 and letter 62.
36 See below, letter 23, note 3.
37 See below, letter 95, note 5.
38 See below, letter 122, note 2.
39 See below, letter 76, note 4.
40 See below, letter 88.

If the history of early modern trade seldom focuses upon individuals, the cause lies more with the limits of surviving sources than with deliberate intellectual longsightedness. Many merchants and their heirs may well have considered business letterbooks as socially, if not morally, incriminating evidence, to be destroyed once their debt-collecting function had been served. London's eighteenth-century statistical records of trade are largely missing, and personal records were lost in myriad fires and shuffles, with the result that relatively little has survived to document that city's mighty preponderance in English trade.[41] If this is true of London's eighteenth-century trade in general, it is even more true of London's trade in the English Atlantic.[42]

Cruttenden's letters provide new evidence and new insights into several aspects of this trade. His business practices were not always what has come to be regarded as typical for the English Atlantic trade at the opening of the eighteenth century. He was not trading safely on commission, but venturing on his own account. He was not an import merchant specializing in bulk shipments of sugar or tobacco, who could watch over the pricing of both sides of his trade and hold balances due to his customers. Unlike some substantial merchants, Cruttenden lacked the political connections that were helpful in trading and in gaining favourable legislation. Some of these differences are rooted in the specialized nature of the drug trade, and this trade preserved most of these peculiarities through the eighteenth century.[43] Some features of his trade derive from the comparatively small scale of his operation, and other features challenge preconceptions about this trade. His business can usefully be analysed in two ways. Firstly, his business connections and general policies on terms of sale, insurance, and smuggling are worth outlining. Secondly, there are a number of telling distinctions between his trade with the West Indies and his trade with New England – distinctions in organization, terms of sale, and nature of returns, which add to the intelligibility and significance of the letters themselves.

Cruttenden's connections were all with British possessions, but there are no

---

41 See A.E.J. Hollaender 'A London Merchant's Letterbook, 1698-1704' *Archives* 3 (1957): 38 and R.G. Wilson *Gentlemen Merchants: The Merchant Community in Leeds, 1700-1830* (Manchester 1971) vii, 1.

42 There is nothing in print for the period 1684 to 1750, that is, between *James Claypoole's Letterbook* ed. Marion Balderston (San Marino, Cal. 1967), ending in 1684, and *John Norton and Sons, Merchants of London and Virginia* ed. Frances Norton Mason, 2nd ed. (London 1968), which begins in 1750. See William I. Roberts III 'Samuel Storke: An Eighteenth Century London Merchant Trading to the American Colonies' *Business History Review* 39 (1965): 147.

43 See S. Stander 'Transatlantic Trade in Pharmaceuticals During the Industrial Revolution' *Bull. Hist. of Med.* 43 (1969): 326-43.

signs that this pattern resulted from government encouragement or restrictions on commerce. He was a small trader operating without living kin abroad and without observable religious connections which could reinforce or replace the trust of kinship.[44] Although he risked sending cargoes to people he did not know, it is not surprising that his trade extended as far as, but no further than, the language he knew and the rule of laws and courts he thought he could understand. He had customers in Jamaica, Antigua, New York, and Madras, but his main trade was to the relatively mature and prosperous colonies of Barbados and Massachusetts.

Cruttenden offered his customers a choice of trading terms, one based upon payment in sterling in London, the other upon prices in colonial currency and payable in the colonies. The first option was his version of the 'commission system' which was becoming increasingly important in the English Atlantic staple trades.[45] Although most commission agents were not giving any credit and were charging 3% on orders and on receipts, Cruttenden charged 10% above wholesale sterling prices for his exports, payable within a year in London. By this method Cruttenden received, warehoused, and sold the customer's commodities, crediting the account with the proceeds minus freight and customs. Cruttenden considered this a reasonable rate for a year's loan of his money, his trouble, and the risk of bad debts. He repeatedly offered this option to all customers who objected to his prices, though relatively few chose this method.[46]

Rather than pay in sterling in London, most of Cruttenden's customers chose to be billed at seemingly higher prices, reckoned in colonial currency and returned in coin (Spanish pieces of eight), bills of exchange, or commodities. Those dealing with him on this basis were able to charge him the current local prices for commodities, coin, and even bills of exchange.[47] The customer usually bore the risks and charges on the relatively compact shipments of drugs and medicines. Cruttenden, who really became the owner of the bulkier colonial commodity returns in the colonies, paid insurance, freight, and customs on these, and gambled on the difference between colonial selling prices and metropolitan buying prices for these colonial goods. His advance

---

44 See Bernard Bailyn 'Communications and Trade: The Atlantic in the Seventeenth Century' *J. Econ. Hist.* 13 (1953): 378-87; Frederick B. Tolles *Meeting House and Counting House* (Chapel Hill 1948) chap. 5.

45 See K.G. Davies 'The Origins of the Commission System in the West India Trade' TRHS 5th series, 2 (1952): 89-107.

46 Davies does not discuss whether the rise of the commission system was at the initiative of the planters or of the London merchants.

47 See below, letters 23 and 81.

on his own exports, the percentage that prices were marked up from whole-sale sterling prices, ranged from 45 to 100% depending upon the colony, the customer, and the kind of goods being ordered. The sterling discount of colonial currency could account for between 20% and all of these increases.[48] The letters also make clear that bad debts were a bigger risk than losses at sea and were insurable only by higher prices. Cruttenden was also lending money without interest, for he did not charge interest on accounts that were several years in arrears. His prices lowered noticeably after the Peace of Utrecht, but appear persistently higher for Massachusetts than for the West Indies because of differences in exchange rates. Goods outside his field of interest and competence were marked up 100% if Cruttenden had to pay cash for them. His advance on drug and medicine prices ranged from 45 to 75%, and Cruttenden insisted that at these rates he did not make 10% on the loan of his money. The sugar trade itself was making 10 to 15% at best, and the prominent clergyman John Tillotson regarded 10% as a moderate rate of profit.[49] One contemporary English provincial merchant, William Stout of Lancaster, withdrew from overseas trade entirely in 1715 after calculating the profits of a Barbados voyage as no more than 10%.[50] At a time when secured investments yielded 5 to 6%, a merchant's return of 10% was regarded as minimal by Cruttenden, yet acceptable by most of his customers.

Cruttenden handled marine insurance in a seemingly casual manner. During the concluding years of the war he did not insure regularly, both be-

[48] Exchange rates altered frequently, and records are sparse.

Year	Price in Local Currency of £100 Sterling*		Boston Price of oz of silver**
	Barbados	Massachusetts	
1710	£133.75	£155.00	8s
1711	£125.42	£146.67	8s 4d
1712	£121.30	£150.00	8s 6d
1713	£120.50	£150.00	8s 6d
1714	£123.50	£153.33	9s
1715		£160.33	9s
1716	£127.50	£162.50	9s 2d–10s
1717	£130.00	£170.00	10s–12s

*Kindly provided by John J. McCusker from his forthcoming *Money and Exchange in Europe and America, 1600-1775: A Handbook* tables 5.2 and 5.3. Figures are annual averages.
**Historical Statistics of the United States, Colonial Times to 1957* (Washington 1960) series z 358. The official price in London was 5s 2d per ounce.

[49] See R.B. Schlatter *Social Ideas of the Religious Leaders, 1660-1688* (Oxford 1940) 213; Richard Grassby 'The rate of profit' 729-31.

[50] Marshall *Autobiography of William Stout* 172

cause rates were above 15%[51] and 'because the Ensurers want insureing.'[52] Cruttenden was lucky, for he reported only one tangle directly related to the war[53] and no cargoes lost in the last four shipping seasons before the peace. After the peace he was less fortunate. A series of losses, beginning in 1714, made it clear that Cruttenden's customers did not readily accept losses either outward or homeward. His attempts to have them pay the wholesale buying price of the lost goods, or even half of that amount, usually met with refusal,[54] and one customer was not heard from in the three remaining years of the letterbook.[55] As insurance rates dropped to the standard peacetime rate of 2½%, Cruttenden informed new customers that he always insured both ways and the customer paid for the insurance outward.[56] With increasing pressure on his prices, he shifted to customer risk both ways or to trade entirely insured. Clearly, it was not just the wealthy merchants who carried their own insurance risks.[57] Cruttenden found insurance uneconomic in wartime and might well have continued to take risks in peacetime as well if he had not been pressed by a series of mishaps.

From his comments upon customs and smuggling, the self-portrait of honest, candid Joseph Cruttenden generally stands. He paid duties and complained, especially about duties on drugs. A shipment of drugs sent to a deceased customer in Jamaica could not be retrieved because the duties would have to be paid a second time on many of the drugs, so they were consigned to a customer in Boston.[58] Smuggling had little to do with his trade, yet his letters show no reticence on the matter. In encouraging a customer in Massachusetts to experiment with returns in pearls he adds 'you may try a few first which may bee gott ashore without Entring, custome ruines all.'[59] These last three words are a refrain throughout the book, but nowhere else are they accompanied by this solution. The only other statement on smuggling was

51 See below, letters 23 and 46.
52 See below, letter 34.
53 A vessel bound for New England was taken by French privateers, retaken by Dutch privateers, and brought into Plymouth, England. Salvage charges were added to customers' accounts, but losses were confined to theft and damage to a trunk while the goods were warehoused. See below, letter 27.
54 See below, letters 73, 107, 111, and 116.
55 Dr Robert Anderson; see below, letter 72.
56 See below, letter 70; for insurance rates see Lucy S. Sutherland *A London Merchant, 1695-1774* (London 1933) 78-9.
57 *Ibid.* 43
58 Habijah Savage; see below, letter 42.
59 See below, letter 76.

made when Thomas Barton thought of returning some juice of liquorice which he did not want. Cruttenden admits: 'I am very glad you did not send the Juice of Liquorish for if you hade the Custome would have been more then tis worth. What wee have here is all run and the Custome saved or else it could never bee sold for the price it is.'[60] He seems to have had very little to do with smuggling, at least in his trade with the English colonies.

Although Cruttenden's trading connections emphasize the unity of the English Atlantic trading empire, the contrasts between his West Indies and New England trade are revealing. Sugar was the difference. As Cruttenden suggested, good quality sugar could always be sold on the London market, and a little could be used by the apothecary himself.[61] Massachusetts returns were another matter, producing different terms and even a different organization of trade.

In Barbados, Cruttenden's business initially revolved around one Conrade Adams, planter, merchant, attorney, and Cruttenden's agent. The terms of their relationship had been arranged as many as fifteen years before the opening of the letterbook,[62] and probably involved a commission of 5%.[63] Adams bought small quantities of drugs and medicines on his own account, but his real service to Cruttenden was in acquiring physicians as customers, forwarding their orders, receiving and delivering shipments and letters on their behalf, making returns to Cruttenden in good sugar, and pursuing debtors. Cruttenden also maintained regular correspondence and duplicate accounts with all his Barbados 'physickmongers'[64] and his advance of 50% apparently included Adams's commission. The wisdom of this correspondence became clear after 1715, when one Barbados customer, Dr William Phillips, began bypassing Adams. This quickly became the way almost all of Cruttenden's Barbados trade was done, and the new advance was 45%. By the end of the letterbook, some Barbados customers were prepared to accept peacetime risks themselves, and so favoured Cruttenden's sterling price option. This now was a 12% mark-up, the original 10% plus 2% for insurance on Cruttenden's exports. Initiative for these changes came from the customers, for Cruttenden had every reason to favour having an agent as long as his prices allowed.

Business with other British West Indian islands was more troublesome and

60 See below, letter 111.
61 See below, letters 31 and 108.
62 See below, letter 47.
63 See below, letter 116. Carl and Roberta Bridenbaugh suggest that a 5% commission was customary; see *No Peace Beyond the Line* (New York 1972) 320.
64 The term is Cruttenden's; see below, letter 4.

less profitable for Cruttenden. The only correspondent left in the Leeward Islands was an ineffective debt collector in a diminishing business. Cruttenden's Jamaica trade was also waning, with most attention upon collecting debts from dead or refractory customers. Cruttenden was corresponding with merchants here, not directly with the indebted physicians or apothecaries, and his were not very effective collectors. Cruttenden linked his one major new customer, Richard Eyton, in a joint account with a Thomas Perkins without their prior knowledge.[65] The prudence of this move by Cruttenden was soon proven by Eyton's death. Compared to his business in Barbados, or in Massachusetts, Cruttenden's trade connections with the Leeward Islands and Jamaica were in very bad repair.

Contrast between Cruttenden's West Indian and New England trade terms is particularly evident from the case of George Jackson, who received a shipment in Barbados and returned to New England before paying Cruttenden. Introducing Jackson to his terms for New England, Cruttenden offered three alternatives: Jackson could pay wholesale sterling prices plus 10% and run all risks; he could pay in goods in London with Cruttenden handling them for him and crediting his account with the proceeds; or he could accept drugs at 75% advance in New England money, to be paid there, with Cruttenden running the risks to England and paying freight. Cruttenden added that most of his returns came in money,[66] which was true of his New England trade. Whatever Jackson's reaction to these suggestions, he did not hurry to accept any of them. A year later he was still trying to decide how to make returns, and five years after that, and after several more letters, Cruttenden arranged to have Jackson sued.[67] Perhaps the 25% increase in prices, most of which had resulted from differences in exchange rates, proved too much for Jackson.

Massachusetts was the colony with which Cruttenden had the most trade, and a trade organized unlike that to the West Indies. Although he had been trading there in the 1690s, most of his New England connections twenty years later were relatively new and active. Some customers were known to be physicians, but there was considerable trade with merchant-apothecaries. Habijah Savage, introduced to trading with Cruttenden by another customer,[68] made returns worth more than £100 sterling per year, or approximately one third of

65 See below, letters 18 and 19.
66 See below, letters 28 and 29.
67 See below, letters 39, 67, and 113.
68 Thomas Barton; see below, letter 13.

Cruttenden's gross annual receipts,[69] and was given 'most-favoured-customer' terms. When other New England customers were paying 75% advances in 1710, Savage was buying at 65%. When other New England customers were exhorted to make returns in coin or bills of exchange, Savage was given the option of making returns in commodities. When all Cruttenden's customers dealt at the pace of a single annual shipment and letter, Cruttenden sent Savage an average of three shipments and letters a year. Cruttenden could not afford an agent in his New England trade, but Savage fulfilled some agency functions. Savage's own apprentice was the only new customer he obtained for Cruttenden,[70] but Savage handled shipments that failed to find their intended customers, and Cruttenden occasionally referred other customers to Savage for particular drugs. A customer having difficulty paying small accounts with bills of exchange was able to pay Savage what he owed Cruttenden.[71] Cruttenden often tried to save on charges by packaging small parcels together and imposing on one customer for delivery to the others. Savage was more willing to do this than was another customer.[72] Peace would force Cruttenden's New England prices down from 75% to as low as 50% advance despite the rising exchange rate, but there could be no change in organization. The very nature of New England returns had already required a lean trade organization.

Relentless insistence upon returns in bullion or bills of exchange from most of his New England customers stands in sharp contrast to Cruttenden's Barbados trade. Bullionism might have been reasonable for bureaucrats and economic theorists, but could a small merchant afford to be a bullionist? Payments in coin or bills of exchange were relatively safe in wartime, as the one would be sent by man-of-war and copies of the other went by several conveyances. Bullion returns were less troublesome for small accounts and better insulated from market reverses than most other commodities. But returns in bullion or bills of exchange were refusals to participate in the possible profits of an Atlantic voyage. Funds that could have been invested in new world commodities for sale in the old were instead being frozen. Cruttenden's insistence upon bills and specie was an insistence that there were no great profits

---

69 Although his acknowledgement of returns was not always full or specific enough to establish values, he did thank correspondents for some £1354.16.0 in the course of 7½ years of trading. Of these adequately mentioned returns, some £358.8.11 (26.4%) was in coin and £428.2.0 (31.6%) in bills of exchange. His returns from Massachusetts were 49% in bills, 31% in coin, and only 20% of the fully recorded returns were in commodities.

70 William Rand; see below, letter 69.

71 Thomas Greaves; see below, letters 75, 94, and 102.

72 Thomas Barton; see below, letter 111.

in importing New England commodities. One transaction with Savage reveals the problem in miniature. Cruttenden sold a bundle of Savage's furs for £8 2s 6d, though Savage had charged him £12 Massachusetts (£8 16s sterling) and the freight and customs charges cost Cruttenden an additional £3.[73] His and other merchants' repeated general laments about losses on returns from New England were based upon experiences like this.[74]

Cruttenden's letters prompt some questions about the advantages of colonial trade under what has come to be called the 'mercantile system.' Did the British imperial network of legal, political, and economic arrangements give advantages to all metropolitan traders? Were the advantages enjoyed by prominent and well-documented English merchants really 'imperial' privileges, or were they just another facet of the advantages of the powerful over the humble? What use were legal appeals from colonial to imperial courts for a trader whose accounts were too small to qualify, and did not equal the attending charges in any case? Were English customs duties on colonial products really a levy on Cruttenden rather than his customers? His caution may have kept his trade within the British empire, but what power did he have over his customers that they did not have over him?

Although Cruttenden's letters can be analysed profitably, they can and do speak for themselves. The plain but artful style of this merchant of limited education spares few words for politics, gossip, or description. His business, of which he was proud, was business. His measure of men was their honesty, reliability, and acumen. Emotion was generally controlled, though his anger escaped the bounds of prudence more often that did his sympathy. His letters not only show the attitudes and problems of a large group of men whom history has been unable to hear, they also present a fairly intimate picture of several intriguing historical survivors who were men of business in the English Atlantic.

The letterbook itself[75] was usually a copybook, recording letters already written, though some entries were altered to suggest that a draft may occasionally

---

73 See below, letter 3.
74 James Claypoole, a London merchant, wrote in 1681, 'I never traded to New England myself and am loath to begin now; there is such great loss by returns'. (Balderston *Claypoole's Letterbook* 63). See C.P. Nettels *The Money Supply of the American Colonies Before 1720* (Madison 1934), especially chap. 3, and Joseph J. Malone *Pine Trees and Politics* (Seattle 1964) chap. 3.
75 'The Letterbook of J.C.' (MS Rawlinson Letterbook 66) was part of Richard Rawlinson's bequest to the Bodleian Library, received in 1756. As the volume bears no marks of conveyance, it is possible that Rawlinson, who was collecting books and manuscripts in London before Cruttenden's

have been made in the letterbook.[76] As no holograph letters have come to light, it is not certain whether the copies are in Cruttenden's hand, or how carefully the copies were made. Lack of paragraphing was common enough, but the scarcity of punctuation, if copied accurately from the original, is relatively uncommon in surviving material of this period.

In editing the text, the 'expanded method' of the *Harvard Guide to American History* has generally been followed.[77] Those of Cruttenden's abbreviations that are still in common use have been retained, without adding punctuation. Some minimal additions to his scanty punctuation have been necessary. These additions have been confined almost entirely to the use of the *semi-colon, which Cruttenden did not use.* Nor did he use square brackets. These have been added to indicate marginalia, and the few editorial additions deemed unavoidable. The latter are also in italic type. Descriptions of people and commodities appear in footnotes, and can readily be traced by consulting the boldface reference numbers in the index. These editorial conventions are intended to make Cruttenden easier to understand, without distorting the unpolished and unpretentious tradesman the reader is about to meet.

death, acquired the volume directly from the estate. See DNB re Rawlinson. Although the letterbook was probably part of a series, nothing else of Cruttenden's was deposited with it or has been discovered elsewhere.

76 For instance, see below, letter 17.

77 (Boston, Mass. 1956) 95-9. Some assistance has also been derived from *The Papers of Benjamin Franklin* ed. L.W. Labaree, 19 vols. (New Haven 1959-) 1: xl-xlv.

ATLANTIC MERCHANT-APOTHECARY:
LETTERS OF JOSEPH CRUTTENDEN
1710-1717

1

To Mr Tho: Barton att Salem
in New England Mar: 3d
1709/10

Sr

yours of November 29th last p Capt Fflint is
before me with the bill of loading for a small
quantity of Sperma Cœti which is not yet come to
hand though the ship arrived at Plimouth a mounth
agoe she is not come about yets, nor know not
when she will, though you gave a very great
price for the sperma Cœti yet if it be fine you
will get mony by it, being now extreamly dear
yet it is somewhat uppon the fall, I never
knew it half the price before it is now att
if its prove very fine and white ye 6d will
be worth 10s att least, whats I make of it
shall give you credit for, and therefore have
charged the Spanish brown and silk handcher
cheifs to you at the prime cost without advance
because I could not stay to see what the Sper
ma Cœti would produce, because the ships wo
uld have been gone. and I think this way
can make no fraction in the accounts. Inclosed
is Invoyce and Bill of lading of your small
order shipt on board Capt Green, which I
wish well to your hands and every way to your
content. I have bought them as well as posble
as I could

Sent by Capt
Green in the
Dolphin. And
Another by —
Capt Miller

The first page of Joseph Cruttenden's letterbook
Courtesy Bodleian Library, Oxford

Mar: 3d 1709/10

SIR

Yours of November 29th last per Capt Flint is before me with the bill of loading for a small quantity of Sperma Coeti[2] which is not yet come to hand though the ship arrivd at Plimouth a mounth agoe she is not come about yet, nor know not when she will. Though you gave a very great price for the Sperma Coeti yet if it be fine you will get mony by it, being now extreamly dear yet it is somewhat upon the fall; I never knew it half the price before it is now att if it prove very fine and white the 6 lbs will be worth 10£ at least. What I make of it shall give you credit for, and therefore have charged the Spanish Brown[3] and silk handchercheifs to you att the prime cost without advance because I could not stay to see what the Sperma Coeti would produce, because the ships would have been gone and I think this way can make no fraction in the account. Inclosed is Invoyce and bill of lading of your small order shipt on board Capt Green, which I wish well to your hands and every way to your content. I have bought them as well as possibly I could. You did not mention which sort of Spanish Brown you would have but it being a thing of so small a price have sent the best. Only this is 28 lbs of the second sort for a specimen, that if you want again you may resolve which to have thereof. The Handchercheifs I have bought as well as I could and hope they will please you. I am sorry for the mistake about the Spicknard[4] but can assure

1 Thomas Barton (1680-1751), son of ship's surgeon John Barton of Salem, became a practising physician in Salem, town clerk, and colonel of the regiment. In 1710, two months after this letter, he married Mary, the grand-daughter of deputy-governor Willoughby (James Savage *A Genealogical Dictionary of the First Settlers of New England* 4 vols. [Boston 1860-2] 1; 134; Malcolm S. Beinfield 'The Early New England Doctor: An Adaptation to a Provincial Environment' *Yale Journal of Biology and Medicine*, 15 [1942-3]: 128-30).

2 Spermaceti is a wax found, in solution, in the head cavities and blubber of the sperm whale. Although widely used in candles, it was also used in ointments for bruises, cuts, pains, coughs, etc. See John Quincy *Pharmacopoeia Officinalis Extemporanea. Or, A Complete English Dispensatory, In Four Parts* 10th ed. (London 1736) 155; John Josselyn *New England's Rarities discovered* (London 1672) 35-6.

3 Spanish Brown is a kind of earth, reddish-brown in colour because of peroxide of iron, which was used as a pigment (OED).

4 Spikenard is the spiky stem of *Nardostachys jatamansi*, a plant of northern India, valued since classical times for the aromatic perfume it yields. In eighteenth-century England it was valued for promoting sweating, strengthening the stomach, dispelling wind, and counteracting poisons (Quincy *Complete English Dispensatory* 176; William Salmon *Pharmacopoeia Londinensis, or the New London Dispensatory* [London 1716] 12; OED). Oil of spikenard was obtained by infusing the nard in Rhine wine, then distilling (Salmon *Pharmacopoeia* 422).

you it lyes at your door for you first gave order for 6 pound of Spicknard not mentioning oyl att all, which I sent you. The next time you sent for oyl Spicknard which I also sent you. The 24 lbs of Lymatura chalybis [5] you also write for, which I can make appear by your invoyce; now I think it is not worth while to send back the steele filings being of so inconsiderable a value. And for the spicknard I would not run the hazzard of the sea till there be peace, and when that will be I see but little likelyhood of; and therefore if you cannot dispose of it, I desire it may lye by for the present, though I see no reason why I should run any risk since it was not my mistake but yours. I hope by the Mast Fleet to hear farthar from you with some returns, which I wish may be in bullion for I can hear of nothing else but what there will be extream loss uppon. The last Sperma Coeti I receivd from New England cost but 4s a pound but it was not refind; the price of it refined is just double of unrefined, for we allways deliver to the refiners as much again as we receive from them.

[*in margin:* Sent by Capt Green in the Dolphin, And Another by Capt Miller]

2

[*13 March 1709/10*]

To Mr Samuell Proctor[1] att Antegua wrote March 13 1709/10 by Mr Vaughan and advised him that received his of the 10 of November last with account that my outstanding Debts there were not yett gott in And adviced him to make all the speed hee could in getting them, that the returnes might bee made by this fleet which hoped would come home earlyer in the yeare than usuall.

5 *Limatura chalybis* are steel filings. Although they were administered internally, they were more often used in the artificial preparation of mineral waters (OED). The internal use was recommended to clear obstructions of the bloodstream and the bowels. Their efficacy was attested to by 'the Twitches they give the stomach sometimes, at their first admission; insomuch as to draw it frequently into a general Contraction, and occasion their Ejectment by Vomit' (Quincy *Complete English Dispensatory* 253).

1 Samuel Proctor was an Antigua merchant of some public note during the governorship of Daniel Parke (1706 10) (CSPC 1708-9, nos. 487 ii, 597 i).

3 MR HABIJAH SAVAGE[1]

London March 3d 1709/10.

SIR

Yours I receivd of Dec 5 last is before me. Am glad to hear the goods shipt for you in Blackmore and Holman are arrivd safe to you and I hope to your content, and can assure you the spice, if you have not disposd of it, is advancd above 20 per Cent of what it cost then, the parliament having laid a very large duty uppon all sorts of Spice.[2] I hope by the mast fleet to receive Effects from you, with a farther invoyce which I shall be willing to comply with if any prospect of advantage appear. Your small barrell of furs is arrivd in Ireland, and there the ship still is and is like to be, with many others some of which have lain there 5 or 6 mounths and dare not stir out for fear of the french that lye on that coast. If she arrive here shall acquaint my self with your man and give him any advice or assistance I am capable of. I fear if the moth were got to the furs before they came from you, they will be worth little if anything before they come here, if they prove never so good they are worth little. I sold the last furs you sent but a few days agoe and got but 8£-2s-6d for them which you charge me 12£ for, beside Freight and customs near 3£ more, so that you see tis dull trading. I wish what you send now may be cheifly in Bullion, which has least loss upon it, and least trouble; but be it what it will I wish it may come safe, for the french are very numerous att sea and take aboundance of our Shipping. This is att present all needfull from   Yours

---

1 Habijah Savage (1674-1746), Boston apothecary and merchant, was the fourth son of Boston merchant-shipowner Thomas Savage. Graduating from Harvard in 1695, Habijah may have been apprenticed to a Boston physician before his MA defence, of Van Helmont's theory of the therapeutic value of magnetism, in 1698. He then established himself as a Boston apothecary and land and office-holder. He married Hannah, daughter of bookseller Samuel Phillips, in 1703, and joined her Old South Church five years later. He was active in the militia and the Artillery Company, rising to the rank of Lieut. Col. in each. He held several public offices in Boston, including three years as a selectman, and represented the town at the General Court in 1717, 1718, and 1732, as well as being a justice of the peace (J.L. Sibley and C.K. Shipton *Harvard Graduates* 16 vols. [Boston 1873-1972] 4: 279-83; John Farmer *A Genealogical Register of the First Settlers of New England* reprinted with corrections by Samuel G. Drake [Baltimore 1969] 254 5; Oliver Ayer Roberts *History of the Military Company of Massachusetts* 4 vols. [Boston 1895-1901] I: 322; *The Diary of Samuel Sewall* 3 vols. [Boston 1878-82] 2: 36, 161; 3: 73n, 140).

2 8 Anne c. 7 imposed new duties on spices for 32 years effective 25 March 1710 (*Statutes* 12: 13).

4 MR CONRADE ADAMS[1]

London March 13th 1709/10 –

SIR

Yours of the 26th of August last I am favoured with, containing an account that you had receivd all the parcells safe by the fleet last year and am greatly concernd about your complaints of the perywiggs, about which I thought I took the best care possible. I wear none my self and so cannot pretend to be a proper judge of them, but I had them made on purpose by a perywiggmaker who I always imploy and who has the caracter of a very honest man. I thought that a likelyer way to have good, than to run the risk of buying those that are ready made for sale, though it seems it proved otherwise. I shewd him your letters and positively asserts every hair in them was new. As to your own parcell of wares I charged the first cost and for the spice it is since advanced to above 20 per cent more than I charged for it. I am sure I took as much if not more care than I should have done for my self. I have alsoe shewn your letter to the man I bought your pickles of. That they should prove bad I cannot but wonder att; I bought such a parcell of him once before and sent by a friend to your Island which proved very good and sold to a good advantage. It was a considerable disapointment to my expectations to have no returns by the last fleet, which came in well and Freight was cheap. I wish it may be so next year, however I am satisfied if you did what you could in the matter. I hope you will not faill of making remittances, if not before yet by the return of this fleet which if it be in goods I request some may be in Capt Potts and the remainder in the Thomas and Elizabeth, Capt Henry Sherbun Commander provided they will take it in uppon as easy terms as any other Good ship will; If not uppon any other good shipp. I hope sugars will not be bought to dear; there will be great loss uppon them if they should, for they are low here. I leave to you to act as you shall Judge will be most for my In-

---

1 An Adams held a plantation in Christchurch parish, Barbados, as early as 1674, and Conrade owned ten acres and twenty-one slaves there in 1679. See Richard Ford *New Map of the Island of Barbadoes* (London 1674) reprinted in Richard S. Dunn 'The Barbados Census of 1680: Profile of the Richest Colony in English America' *William and Mary Quarterly* 3rd ser., 26: 16-17; J.C. Hotten *The Original Lists of Persons of Quality* ... (London 1874) 473. Conrade Adams had lived in Salem, Massachusetts, for a time, but was doing business from Barbados with Samuel Sewall of Boston in the 1690s (C.P. Nettels *The Money Supply of the American Colonies before 1720* [Madison 1934] 83n; *Letterbook of Samuel Sewell* 2 vols. [Boston 1886-8] 1: 141, 246-7). Planter, attorney, and merchant, Adams was Cruttenden's Barbados agent. See above, p. xxi. Also see *Acts of the Privy Council of England, Colonial Series* ed. W.L. Grant and J. Munro, 6 vols. (London 1908-12) 2 no. 1201.

terest, which I doe not in the least question but you will doe. I could have wisht for more invoyces this year for I think it strange to miss a year and send nothing to Barbados which I doe not remember I every did before since I first began to deal with your brother. I know there has been great quantitys of medicines and druggs shipt to your Island by this fleet, and it has been no small concern to me that none of them hath fallen to my lot. Though you write there is no incouragement, yet I am very unwilling to lose that small interest I hope I have there and cannot but think if you would converse a little among the physickmongers of yours but you might procure some more business. I am sure no one of the trade is more capable and ready to it than my self. I therefore again request you would procure what business you can for me against next which if it please god to spare life you may depend uppon receiving. I have discoursed with Mrs Potter about what you writt, but Cannot satisfye her about it nor have not received any mony of her; she promised me to write to you about her objections which I hope she has done. I would be glad the matter were issued² and wish I had not advised in the matter but cannot help it now, but will doe anything I can to assist you in the matter. I am glad you have made so good a step towards getting in Dr Houghs debt,³ and wish you success in the remainder. I am really concernd for the mans circumstances and would shew him any reall kindess but still must have a regard to my self and family and I am sure he ever had a pennyworth for his penny in all he had of me, and indeed I cannot afford to lose so large a sume. I think there is considerably above a 100£ due deducting that sum you mention you have securd viz: 137£ 7s 6d You know I have born the fategues of the war and have met with severe loses. I would therefore hope that for the future, (by your assistance in promoting my dealings) in some measure to retreive it which I shall be very glad to doe. This is all att present from   Yours

JC

[*in margin* Sent by the Samuell, Capt Brookes and another by the Mary, Capt Holliday]

---

2 Issue, in the sense of end, close, or termination, was a noun, according to OED, the verb meaning to come as proceeds or revenue.
3 Two years later, Adams succeeded in collecting some, but not all, of this debt. See below, letter 31.

5 CAPT JAMES PITTS[1]

Lond March 2 1709/10

I hoped to have received the Bill from you by these last shipps that came in which you promised to send last year by the Mast Fleet. I wait in hopes I shall receive it by the next Mast Fleet. You know it has been a great while and the goods were bought with ready money and noe advance upon them and therefore will not beare soe long Credit. Your shipp David and Joseph[2] is comeing to New England againe; all her last voyage is Marooned againe for Eton was broke before her arrivall and the Masts would not pay half the Freight. Soe Mr Waterhouse[3] upon his owne whim shipt them againe in the same Ship for Lysbon where they will not sell and there Capt Arnold[4] has left them, a perticuler account of which hee will give you. Mr Waterhouse has never yett rendred any account nor whether ever hee will I know not; nor have I received a penny of him since you were here; what he designes I know nott. As I formerly hinted, if you know any person that you judge substantiall if you can recommend them to me it shall bee complyed with, and kindly received by Sir   Yours   JC

Sent by Capt Emerson and by Mr Rand

1 A Captain James Pitts of Boston, Mass., merchant, was registered as part owner of the new sloop *Adventure*, on 16 October 1710. Co-owners were Lt. Col. Thomas Savage and Richard Hill (State House, Boston, Massachusetts Archives 7: 380). Cf. Charles M. Andrews and Frances G. Davenport *Guide to the Manuscript Materials ... in the British Museum, in Minor London Archives, and in the Libraries of Oxford and Cambridge* (Washington 1908) 410.
2 Cruttenden was part owner of this vessel, hence his interest in its profitability. Pitts, Waterhouse, and perhaps Eton were shareholders with Cruttenden, who presumably contributed cargo or provisions several years earlier. See below, letter 10. Bernard and Lotte Bailyn's *Massachusetts Shipping, 1697-1714* (Cambridge, Mass. 1959) 56-73 discusses transatlantic shareholding.
3 Probably Mr David Waterhouse, a leading London merchant in the New England trade. See Byron Fairchild *Messrs William Pepperrell: Merchants of Piscataqua* (Ithaca, NY 1954) 47 and Nettels *Money Supply* 145n.
4 Captain of the *David and Joseph*; see below, letter 10.

6 TO MR THOMAS LITTLE OF PLYMOUTH[1]

Mar:- 9 1709/10

SIR

Haveing this opertunity per a Freind I could not satisfyce my self without paying my respects to you in a line or 2. I hope to heare from you by the Mast fleet which are expected in 6 weekes or 2 months and shall bee glad of a good large Invoyce; for tho I have mett with as small incourgement as most have done, yet am still willing to venture againe hoping some time or other things will bee better. Shall adde noe more but etc.   JC

7 TO MR WILLIAM WEAVER[1] ATT BARBADOS

Mar 3 1709/10

SIR

Inclosed is a letter to your father, the contents whereof you see. All I request of you is that you would satisfye Mr Joseph Ward which is that Mr John Brown (if there bee more then one of that name in your Island) that was over here in England about 6 yeares agoe. His wife, your father tells me, kept a publick house. I doubt not but you know the man. when hee was here he contracted a debt to me of about 20£ which he promised to returne by the next fleet but could never gett a line from him since. And by Mr Joseph Ward (who I empowered as my Attourney to receive it) I understand hee denys the Debt and offers to make oath that hee never knew me or hade any dealing with me. Now I admire att the impudence of the man for hee was frequently

---

1 Thomas Little (1674-1712) was born in Marshfield, Plymouth colony. He graduated from Harvard in 1695 and settled in Plymouth about 1700. Here he was a merchant, ship owner, real estate speculator, and office holder, but was best known as a gentleman physician who did his own surgery and drug dispensing (James Thacher *American Medical Biography* [Boston 1828] 18; Sibley *Harvard Graduates* 4: 252-3; Massachusetts Archives 7: 176, 181, 391).

1 A Weaver, perhaps the father of this correspondent, was part owner of a Barbados plantation in St George Parish in 1674 (Ford, *Map of the Island of Barbadoes*). A William Weaver was registered as owning 100 acres and thirty slaves in the same parish five years later and received custody of two convicted participants in Monmouth's rising in 1685 (Hotten *Original List of Persons of Quality* 329, 461).

att my house and dined with me and I bought a parcell of Aloes[2] of him to the value of 62£ 3s which I paid him for and have sent over his receipt which he gave me with his owne hand. Now certainely hee must bee the most impudent person liveing to deny his owne hand. If I hade lost 5 times as much money providentially I could have borne it patiently but this is plaine cheating, and therefore if hee bee able I am resolved to try to make him willing. I have proved my debt before the Lord Major[3] by my hand that the goods were delivered to him and I thinke your laws must bee very defective if they will not oblige him to pay it. I hope you'l excuse this trouble which I hade not given you but for the reasons mentioned and your father assured me he doubted not you would readyly comply with. Shall adde noe more but with etc.   JC

8 TO MR JOSEPH WARD ATT BARBADOS

Mar: 13 1709/10

SIR

Yours of Sept the 4th 1709 per Sophia Packett boat[1] I have received and note the contents. I cannott but admire att the Impudence of Mr Browne (unlesse by the way there bee more of that name then one and you have gone to the wrong [one] but Mr Weaver can satisfye you fully in the matter for tis that Browne that he recommended to his father) that hee should deny his debt and say hee never knew me when hee was frequently att my house and dined with me. And to satisfye you that hee knew me I have here inclosed sent a receipt with his owne hand writeing of his name to it for 62£-3s-I paid him for a parcell of Aloes I bought of him, for which by the way hee was forward

---

2 Aloes is the juice of the fleshy leaves of the aloe plant native to East and South Africa, but cultivated in the West Indies, Barbados producing the best quality. It was valued as a purgative, but modern cautions include the fact that it induces piles, causes severe griping and possible kidney damage, and can poison children (Quincy *Complete English Dispensatory* 78; M. Grieve *A Modern Herbal* 2 vols. [New York 1931] 1: 26-9; W.W. Bauer *Potions, Remedies and Old Wives' Tales* [Garden City, NY 1969] 210).

3 Lord Mayor of London

---

1 The *Sophia* was one of Edmund Dummer's packets, here sailing as the fifty-fourth clockwise North Atlantic service. The *Sophia* left Barbados for the western Caribbean on 18 November, and brought her mail into Clovelly on 28 January following. This seems to be the only reference to the packet service being used by any of Cruttenden's correspondents, supporting suspicions that it was considered too expensive. On the packet service, see James Hamilton St John 'Edmund Dummer and His West India Packets' *University of Iowa Studies in the Social Sciences* 11 (1941): 125-46; John Haskell Kemble 'England's First Atlantic Mail Line' *Mariner's Mirror* 26 (1940): 33-54, 185-98.

enough for he would scarce stay till the time agreed for the money. I have asked advice of a Lawyer here who says his swearing hee owes noe such debt cannot bring him off for if mens swearing they owe their creditors nothing will bee sufficient to Balance their accounts you would have it done every day; besides his owne hand writeing must cost him certainely if your laws are good for any thing. And farther to satisfye you he had dealeing with me he left a Debenture in the Custome house for me to receive for him which I did and have given him creditt for it in his account. I have lost manny a hundred pound and if this were providentially lost I would not value it but I hate to bee cheated by a Rascall that has receivd such kindnesses from me. And therefore my desyre is that you bee first well satisfied of the right man (which Mr Weaver can easly do and therefore I have inclosed a letter to him as all-soe one from his father to desyre his assistance in the matter) and of his circumstances and if hee bee able arrest him forthwith and prosecute him with all the vigour you can. I am told you are in the wrong for suffer him to swear he owed nothing whereas you should forthwith have arrested him haveing a full power to doe it and the debt authentickly proved before the Lord Major. If he has sworne it, certainely produceing his own hand will prove him perjured and then you may bring him to the Pillory; I cannot but beleive, if you have any degree of Justice to bee hade among you, but you may recover the debt and force him to pay all the Charges. I leave the matter to you etc. Please to give my Service to your Brother and remind him of his conditionall promise to make tryall of me when he has any orders in my way which I am sure I can and will furnish him with as cheap as any one in London. You may before wittnesse ask him [*Browne*] if that bee not his owne hand which I cutt out of my receipt booke which is the reason of that writeing on the back side please to take care you doe not loose it for I cannott but [*in margin*: Thinke that must bee of great use if you come to a tryall. This is the need full from etc.   JC]

9 MR HABIJAH SAVAGE

London June 27 1710

SIR

Yours of February 23 is before me which inclosed a bill of lading for 300 peices 8[1] which came to my hands safe for which I return you hearty thanks;

---

1 A piece of 8 was a Spanish silver coin having an English sterling equivalent of 4s 6d in 1703 (Public Record Office, London, CO 5/1262, fols. 150-1). This value, for a full 17 pennyweight Saville, Mexican, or pillar piece of 8, was established as the legal exchange rate in 1708, though the colonists consistently paid more (Nettels *Money Supply, passim*).

it came to a tolerable markett but not so high by 3d an ounce as last year, but however I cannot but judge it better than any sort of goods as things are att present. Also received your invoice for an other parcell of goods, Invoyce and bill of lading of which comes inclosed by Capt Bond in the ship Partridge which I wish well to your hand and every way to your content which I have to the utmost indeavourd. This ship sayling sooner then the others designing to goe North about goes away sooner than expected so must defer my larger writing to the next shipps which will sayl in 14 days and perhaps may reach you as soon as this. What I can spare time for, and what is absolutely needfull is to hint to you, that I have complyd with your desire and charged but 65£ perCent advance on all the things now sent (except those few directly out of my way, and bought with ready mony and no advance uppon them) but att 65£ perCent advance and none att all on the petty charges which have made all distinct though I must say I can see no incouragement so to doe, for the druggs being the far greater part being bought with ready mony and no advance on many of them, and very little uppon any (none higher than your self could have bought them were you here) and to advance but 65 per cent allowing for insurance which runs high and the very great loss upon all returns, I am sure brings it down to very little. Besides losses must be expected this war time, which if one should happen the profit of many years would be gone att once. I could lay out my mony in 20 sort of commoditys and send to New England for which I could have much more than Cent per Cent advance, can see no reason why the same allowance should not be made on my goods as others provided they be bought as well and not advanced on. I have settled my book as you make it that there can be no mistake about it I have sent no spice for if you were dissatisfyed before I cannot pretend to please you now, and what ever you hint of there having them cheaper charged, I must begg your pardon in suspending my beleif of it, for I bought them as cheap as possibly I could and cheaper by 20 perCent then I can buy them now. I am well assured att that time none could buy them cheaper if they were as good there has been so large a tax layd uppon all spice this year that has raisd it so much as discouraged me from sending it. I had not room to put up all the 12 grosse of vials and could get no dryed liquorish[2] nor good Juniper berrys[3] so have sent but 7 lbs of them but it may be by that time the next ships sayle

---

2 Liquorice, the root of a shrub native to southern Europe and Southwestern Asia, was highly regarded for throat and chest complaints and widely used to mask the taste of other medicines (Quincy *Complete English Dispensatory* 149; Salmon *Pharmacopoeia* 9).

3 Unripe juniper berries were distilled to produce an oil which was diuretic, a stomach strengthener, and effective in cases of jaundice, dropsies, and infections (Quincy *Complete English Dispensatory* 143). William Salmon claimed additional merits for the berries, seeing them as effective against plague and fevers, venomous bites, and stones (*Pharmacopoeia* 120-1).

may gett the rest and send with them remaining 3 grosse of vials, and it may be some small quantity of spice to supply your present necessity, till I can hear from you again. The druggs are the best of every thing except the Juniper berrys than which there are none better. I intreat you to excuse brevity for the reason above mentioned shall add no more but remain with hearty service remain etc.   JC

[*in margin:* Sent by the Partridge Capt Bond]

10 COPPY OF WHAT SENT IN CAPT BOND ETC.

SIR

Am now arrived to the 1st day of August and this serves to inclose a second Bill of Ladeing and Invoyce of those things shipt you in Capt Bond as allsoe a Bill of Loading and Invoyce of a small case shipt for you on Capt Partis of the Liquorish and remainder of the violls which I writt you word I could not gett then, since which I met with a hundred weight of fine dry Liquorish; you find it charged but half the price that the 12 lbs was before sent but that cost me the price I charged for it and I did not gett a farthing either by one or other. You will find in the Case a small box directed for Mr Thomas Greaves[1] att Charles Towne which I desyre the favour of you to deliver to him upon demand he paying what you judge proportionable for Freight etc. I have advised him of it. I did endeavour allsoe to have sent the Juniper Berrys but could gett none good the season for them will now quickly be heare and by the first conveyance will supply you with them. I proposed to my self allsoe to have sent to you some Spice but upon enquireing find the price soe prodigiously advanced that it discouraged me to venture for feare you should be Frighted att it. Pepper which I last charged you but 17d for is now 3s-4d a pound and all spice extremely dear tho not quite soe much if I can meet with any opertunity to gett any upon more reasonable termes you may possibly have some yett I would, if I knew how, act most for your satisfaction and advantage. I have concidered what you write about oyl of Turpentine[2] and cannot see any incouragement att 2s 6d a Gallon it is as dear as can buy it for

1 See below, letter 11, note 1.
2 Oil of Turpentine is produced by distillation of common turpentine, though that of Venice and especially Chios was more highly prized and priced; Oil of Chios Turpentine retailed for 1s per ounce in 1681 (William Salmon *Synopsis Medicina* 2nd ed. [London 1681] catalogue of prices). Oil of turpentine was valued in preparing medicines because it dissolved gums and was easily infused with perfume essences. It was also reputed to cure 'Wounds of the nervous Parts to a wonder' (Salmon *Pharmacopoeia* 417-18). Also see Thomas Healde *The New Pharmacopoeia of the Royal College of Physicians of London* (London 1788) 70-1 and *Ency. Brit.* 27: 481-2.

heare and tis such a penetrating thing that tis odds but a third part is leak't out. I remember I once hade some come home and there was extreame losse in it. If Turpentine itself bee cheap I had rather have that or fish oyle; if you could meet with any Sperma Coeti It would turne to a good account. Furrs are very cheap and Dear Skinns cheaper than last yeare by 20 per Cent tho after all if it may bee procured had rather have it in Silver: if this comes times enough and you ship any goods for me I would bee glad if you shipt it on the David and Joseph, Capt Arnold because I have a part of that ship. I leave it to you to act for me as for yourself and after all the small misunderstandings hope to continue my Correspondance with you as long as wee live and can assure you if you think I designe otherwise you much mistake me for I greatly value your Correspondance and shall always do soe and endeavour to consult your interest and satisfaction to the uttmost of my power who am etc.   Yours

JC

11 TO MR THOMAS GREAVES[1] OF CHARLES TOWNE IN NEW ENGLAND

London Aug: 1: 1710

SIR

Yours of Jan 25 last is before me contents of which have observed and this serves to inclose Invoyce of your very small order, which was soe small that I was afraid it would bee lost sent by it self and therefore I have put it up in a Parcell of goods for Mr Habijah Savage; they are in a small box directed on the topp for you which I have desyred to deliver to you upon demand and doubt not but hee will. What small proportion of Freight he demands you must pay but it can't bee much. As to the Sal Viperarum[2] it is a[s] cheap as ever I bought it and the price I allways give for it when prescribed; such a volatile thing as that must bee decayed in all that time therefore to expect to returne it cannott bee just or reasonable. I am well assured it never came

1 Thomas Greaves (1683-1747), physician and judge, was son of Thomas Greaves, physician, magistrate, and Andros supporter. Young Thomas graduated from Harvard in 1703 and became a highly regarded physician and teacher of apprentice physicians (Sibley, *Harvard Graduates* 5: 211-16; Timothy Cutler *Good and Faithful Servant* [Boston 1747] *passim*; J.M. Toner *Contributions to the Annals of Medical Progress in the United States, Before and During the War for Independence* [Washington 1874] 23; Sewall *Diary 3:* 87, 119, 139, 210, 254, 398). Greaves was a relatively new customer for Cruttenden, and his orders were on the limited scale of a dispensing physician.

2 *Sal viperarum* is a volatile salt derived from burning vipers. It was considered as giving relief in apoplexy, palsies, mental disorders, asthma, etc., and especially useful for all skin ailments (Quincy *Complete English Dispensatory* 339).

cheaper to any person in New England then the price I charged it att; the dose is small and that answeares the dearnesse of it; however if you returne it I will endeavour to dispose of it for you but shall not take it upon my owne account. As to your larger Invoyce you mention shall if receive it comply with it and forward to you by the next good Conveyance and shall gladly settle a farther correspondance with you; And shall always take care to supply you with what is good and reasonable or any Freind or aquaintance you can recommend me to that you know is substantiall. As for the returne you may send it in the man of warr that convoys the Mast fleet. In Forreigne Silver is best, all Comoditys being low and troublesome and the sume soe small it will not bee worth your while to trouble yourself to buye them. Shall add no more but remaine etc.

[*in margin*] Shipt on board the Nicholson, Capt Partis by whom this letter goes and a Coppy of ditto per Capt [*blank*] in the [*blank*] Note: I wrote to him againe Aug 25, 1712 by Capt Savage and advised him had Shipt his things againe in Capt Whellan and hade paid for Salvage 14s-6 which made his bill: 4-18-6]

12 MR WILLIAM LITTLE[1] OF BOSTON NEW ENGLAND

London Aug 1 1710

SIR

Yours of January 30 last is before me, and observe the contents. And to passe by your Complyment which I thinke above my deserts and ability to returne and therefore shall content myself onely by telling you I am well pleased if my sincere endeavours to serve my Freinds in your Country have mett with any acceptation and that I am still ready and willing to serve you or any Freind of yours to the uttmost of my power. I received the 32½ ozs Silver by Capt Peal the produce whereof you see in the Inclosed Invoyce. I have sent all the Bookes in the Catalogue, with the Drops and Scutcheons[2] which wish may prove to your content, which I have endeavoured; I tryed very much among the Booksellers to gett them as cheap as I could and found by all of

---

1 William Little (b. 1692?) was the fifth of Isaac Little's six sons and younger brother of Thomas Little, Plymouth physician and regular customer of Cruttenden (*Mayflower Descendant* 24 [1922]: 1, 2, 6); also see below, letters 38, 46, 112.

2 Scutcheons, or escutcheons, are nameplates, backplates for key holes, etc. 'Drops and scutcheons' were probably drawer or cupboard door handles with backplates. See below, letter 46.

these they were a choice collection of New an[d] valuable Bookes. I have charged them as they cost and in the drops and Scutcheons have saved you a dozen shillings att least by bespeakeing[3] them of the maker and soe hade them cheaper, by soe much then could have hade them of the Shopps. The Bookes are all the best Edition I thinke; As for the other Bookes mentioned in the letter that you proposed some Bookeseller to send, I proposed it to 2 or 3 of my aquaintance but could not find they were willing to comply; they objected they were very dear books and such as were ready money. You see by the inclosed bill of parcelles I have disbursed for you 4£-15s Sterling more then the produce of your Silver which you may returne per the Man of warr or by Bill as you thinke best. I have charged noe Commissions, if my Marketting please you and you thinke I deserve anything I leave it to you to act as you please; And if you can bee servicable in promoting my Interest with any persons that deale in my way I should account it a favour; I am sure noe one can supply them cheaper. There is one Dr Creed or such a name I have heard well of if you can make any interest with him (if you judge him substantiall) I should thinke it a great favour, you that live upon the spott must know in a great measure who are the fittest persons to deale with. I putt up your goods in a Trunk as judgeing that might bee usefull for other ocasions; you will find a paper of Nayls put up to make any letters on the lid you shall have a mind to. Inclosed is Bill of Loading as well as Invoyce. Pray when you have opertunity give my Service to your Brother att Salem[4] from whom I received noe letter by this last fleet but hope I shall by the next. [*in margin:* as to your comoditys they are mostly Dull; if you could meet with any Sperma Coeti tis much wanted and would turne to account if not exceed 10 or 12 shillings a pound. In oyle Traine oyle[5] will doe pretty well. Furrs are very low Turpentine may doe tollerably well if bought cheap.] This with hearty Service is all the needfull From Sir

Sent by the Nicholson, Capt Partis allsoe a Copy by [*blank*]

3 Bespeakeing, arranging for (OED)
4 Mistake for Plymouth; see above, note 1.
5 Train oil, from the blubber of northern whales, was used in oiling wools for carding and in other commercial processes, and was burned to provide artificial light.

13 TO MR THOMAS BARTON ATT SALEM IN NEW ENGLAND

Aug: 1 1710

SIR

Yours of January – last is before me and the Silver in the Reserve came safe to my hands and to a tollerable markett better then any goods would have done except sperma Coeti, I sold it for 5s 5d per oz.[1] Allsoe received your Account Current But I cannott comply with it as to your chargeing me for Freights and dutys and petty charges tis what I never heard of and what you never mentiond to my knowledge. Mr Savage never desyred any such thing. As to the Lymat Chalibis and Spicknard I have I thinke sufficiently answeared in my last letter and since the mistake was yours I cannot see reason why I should stand to the loss of it for I am possitive you directly sent for each of them; I will doe any thing you shall desyre that is reasonable and if you send it back will take it againe, but will not run the risques of it. As to what you write about the Hungary water[2] If you had bottles as big again before (which I doe not remember) yet it is now as Deare againe, Rosemary Flowers[3] being 6 times as Dear as they were 2 yeares agoe, the hard winter having destroyed it all allmost and I am possitive of it cannot buy such for the money now as I sent you last: however I desyre you to dispose of them as you can and am willing to make what reasonable allowance you shall desyre. I have inclosed your Account Current as I have settled it in by Booke which is not much different from yours and you see the Ballance is 45-18-¾. Youl remember the last parcell came since your account was made, I hope wee shall

---

1 This is 3d above the official price in England. Barton was using Cruttenden's sterling price option at this time. See above, p. xix, note 48.

2 Hungary water, or 'That noble, reviving Cephalic Liquor, called the *Queen of Hungary's Water*' (Thomas Short *Medicina Britannica* 3rd ed. [Philadelphia 1751] 245), was wine infused with rosemary flowers. Used as a medium for other medicines and as a cold remedy, it was particularly valued for dislodging hardened wax from the ears as well as a remedy for 'dumb palsy,' loss of speech, and 'falling sickness' (Quincy *Complete English Dispensatory* 72, 367; Healde *New Pharmacopoeia* 163, 320; Nicholas Culpeper *Culpepper's English Physician and Complete Herbal* [London c. 1695] 313).

3 Rosemary, a Mediterranean shrub, produces flowers, the oil from which was valued as a perfume base and a medicine. The oil was used in ointments or drunk in a decoction, and the leaves were dried, smoked with tobacco, or crushed and moistened to make a poultice for the temples. Rosemary was considered helpful for colds, dropsies, headaches, toothache, and nervous disorder, and as a decongestant (Culpeper *English Physician* 323; Quincy *Complete English Dispensatory* 72; *A Collection of … Receipts in Cookery, Physick and Surgery* 2nd ed. [London 1719] 132; Grieve *Modern Herbal* 2: 681-3; according to Josselyn, it could not be grown in New England [*New England's Rarities* 89]).

have noe further complaints or difference but that all may goe on Smoothly; I am sure I desyre it may and doe once for all promise you that you shall [*have all?*] incouragement you can desyre in Corresponding with me. I have noe reason or cause to complaine (nor never did) of your pay which is very good besides I thinke my self under a further obligation to you for recommending to Mr Savage; and therefore you may depend on it I shall never disagree to anything you shall reasonably desyre. I made the most I could of your Sperma Coeti which was 28s a pound tho it was very good yet it was not fitt for use but must bee refined and the refineing is as much as if it had been worse, but it turned to a pretty good account; I wish you could meet with more of it, I know nothing you can send that will advance soe much tho I suppose it cannot hold long att such a price. I shall adde noe more but remain   Yours   JC

14 TO MR GEORGE GREEMES ATT BARBADOS

Dec: 20 1710

SIR

I received both yours bearing date the 1 of August 1710: with your inclosed Invoyce for Druggs and Medicines, And must onely informe you I never received a line from you last year. If I had received any Invoyce from you you might have depended on the things for I would not have disapoynted you, therefore for the future you would do well to send by 2 or 3 ships for there is danger of miscarryage this warr time and when it will end God onely knows. This serves to Inclose an Invoyce and Bill of Loading for 2 small cases conteining your whole Invoyce shipt on board Capt John Swan in the London Friggott who is a good Ship and sayles the greatest part of the way with the Jamaica Convoy; I consulted with Mr Hoyle about it who approved well of my Shipping it upon him. I concider your disapoyntment last year and that the Barbados Fleet would not sayle this 3 months and therefore upon the whole concidering what a disapoyntment it might prove to you, with the consent of Mr Hoyle, have sent them by this Conveyance. I wish them safe to your hands and every way to your content and satisfaction and shall bee glad to continue a yearly correspondance with you and doe once for all promise you shall have very fayr and Candid dealing from me: I have I hope soe contrived the matter that noe manner of damage can come haveing put all the Liquids in one case and the Dry in another; and for the prizes I have gone as low in every perticuler as I could have done hade you been here upon the

Spott. The Pul è Chel b/is Comp[1] I have charged 10s. an ounce for whereas formerly use to charge but 8s an ounce but the reason is Bezoars[2] are att such an extravagant price and like still to bee dearer, if they cannot bee sold for lesse then 10s nor well for that, wee sell it here now for 12 shillings an ounce and often for more; Bezoars are worth very neare 5 pound an ounce. I thought fitt to give you this one hint that you might have noe suspicion that I would in the least attempt to impose upon you, but give you all incouragement possible to continue a farther correspondance; every thing sent are good and hope they will come Soe to you. I have discoursed with Mr Hoyle about accepteing your Bill; he has promised after your Sugars are sold and the other Bills you have drawne on him satisfyed if there bee enough left he will pay the whole of my Bill if not will pay as farr as it goes; he is unwilling to sell the Sugars till toward the, Spring hopeing they will then bear a little better price for att present they are extremely low: I shall if please God to continue life give you a farther account by the Fleet of all that is done in the matter. The Fleet talk of sayleing about March: There was a little roome left in one of the cases which I filled up with half a Grosse of violls more then your order which suppose can bee noe disapoyntment to you

15 FOR MR CONRADE ADAMS ATT BARBADOS

London Dec: 20 1710

SIR

I am favoured with both yours of June 6 last per Capt Bartlett and Waldic with Inclosed Invoyce from Dr William Phyllips which I have complyed with

1 *Pulvis è chelis cancrorum compositus,* or Gascoigne's powder, was made of ground pearls, crabs' eyes, red coral, amber, harts horn, black tops of crab claws, and oriental bezoar, the most valued ingredient. This powder was esteemed as able to resist plague and allay fevers, and was especially regarded as an antidote to poisons. In 1678 Boston physician Thomas Thacher warned, in the first medical broadside printed in America, that too many hot cordials, including Gascoigne's powder, can cause 'Phrenzies' in smallpox sufferers (reprinted in Maurice B. Gordon *Aesculapius Comes to the Colonies* [Ventnor, NJ 1949] 112-13). In the course of the eighteenth century, this type of medicine will be driven from the pharmacopoeias. In 1716, however, Salmon still regarded it highly, though he warned against adulteration of bezoars (*Pharmacopoeia* 183, 557). Quincy, writing in 1736, is doubtful of the value of Gascoigne's powder (*Complete English Dispensatory* 179-80).

2 Bezoars, or bezoar stones, were concretions from the stomachs of ruminants, especially wild goats of Persia (oriental bezoar stones). Composed of hair, vegetable fibres, and acids, they were valued as an antidote to poison and to check bleeding (Salmon *Pharmacopoeia* 183; Quincy *Complete English Dispensatory* 179-80; *Ency. Brit.* 11: 418; 12: 162).

upon your termes and have forwarded to you by this first Conveyance viz Capt John Swan who will[1] sayle with the Jamaica Convoy which I wish safe to your hands and to his full satisfaction. Inclosed is Invoyce and Bill of Ladeing of the sayd Parcell. I hope I have done everything for the content and satisfaction of Dr Phyllips and what may incourage a farther Correspondance with him which I shall bee very foreward to doe. I hope I have taken such care that there can bee noe damage and will every way please him. Alsoe were favoured with yours of June 20 with advice of your Shipping for me 20 hoggsheads on Capt Potts and Sherburne which I allsoe received together with your further invoyces for yourself and Mr Jemmett which, God spareing life, shall not fayle to forward to you per the Fleet which hope to sayle early in the spring. The Sugars in Capt Potts received conciderable Damage by oversayle the ship was streined and tooke in water; I lost neare 18 cwt of Sugar but hope to have some allowance from the owners when the matter is made up; some people had all their Sugar gone. That in Sherburne came very well but both to a very low markett; I sold them but for 25s 6d per long hundred which was a very great losse but however I desyre to bee thankfull they came soe safe home att all this hazzardous time of warr, which is still like to bee continued. Wee have noe prospect here att all of any peace and therefore wee must beare it as well as wee can.   Yours etc   JC

16 [*Conrade Adams*]

London Feb: 22 1710/11

SIR

This serves to informe you further that I have Shipt on Capt Potts with the Fleet your owne Invoyce and allso that for Mr Jemmett and inclosed is Invoyce and Bill of loading of both Parcells; your owne goods are all intirely by themselves in the smallest Chest No. 3 onely there is 10 pounds of Tin which belongs to Mr Jemmett which was putt in to fill it up which please to deliver to him. I have taken all possible care in your owne things and Mr Jemmetts and wish them safe to your hands and to your full contentment as well as his and that they may lay the plattforme of a farther and more conciderable dealing with him which I hope you will endeavour as allsoe any other persons you can procure who am Sir etc.   Yours   JC

---

1 'With' in the manuscript

17 TO DR WILLIAM PHYLLIPS IN BARBADOS

Dec: 20 1710 –

SIR

Your Invoyce for Druggs and Medicines under Covert of Mr Conrade Adams is come safe to hand the Contents whereof I have forwarded to you by Capt John Swan which heartyly wish well to you and to prove to your content. I have perticulerly taken care to observe your order about them and have sent the best of every sort: I thinke myself bound to pay my respects to you in this manner and to assure you I shall bee ambitious of corresponding yearly with you and shall allways take extraordinary care in every thing to oblige you. I doe promise noe one in London shall bee able to deale more candidly by you then myself and shall bee glad of any opertunity of satisfying you how ready I am to serve you: Shall adde noe more but remaine with etc. (Yours JC) I could have been gladd you had been a little more perticuler in your orders about the stills[1] as to their dimensions; I have sent them of 2 sizes and hope they will please you. I desyre for the future you will bee very exact [*in margin:* in your orders and you shall find me as exact in my complyance with them who am Sir   Yours etc]

18 TO MR RICHARD EYTON ATT JAMAICA

Janry: 3: 1710/11 –

SIR

I received both yours of June 12 1710 with a large Invoyce of Druggs and Medicines which you write you had agreed with a Doctor to take off upon Arrivall there att Cent per Cent advance; I thinke you would have done well to have mentioned who the Doctor was[1] that I might have made inquiry what Character I could have heard of him which was a great omission. However I have concidered of the matter and tho the Quantity bee great and come to great deal of money and most of them Druggs wherein is noe advantage yet I have adventured to put them and forwarded them to you by this Conveyance vizt Captaine Madden in the Robert and Francis which sayles with good

---

1 These must have been apothecary's stills in view of the way Cruttenden filled the order, not sugar equipment. This is evidence of the physician who is his own apothecary to the extent of distilling oils, etc.

1 Apparently the customer was a Dr Tredway; see below, letter 86.

Convoy and in the Fleet which I wish safe to your hands and to your Freinds content, inclosed is Bill of Loading and Invoyce. I have sent everything of the Best and the prices as low as possible of two or 3 of the perticulers I have sent a smaller quantity then was ordered by reason of the extraordinary dearnesse of them as the Camboog.[2] And the Mellilett[3] the quantity was soe large I could not spare soe much soe have sent but 50 lbs which to bee sure must bee enough to serve him till another year when he may have what quantity he pleases. He allsoe writes for Plague water[4] and Surfeit water;[5] now wee comonly reckon them the same but have sent one Bottle of Red Surfeit water which is an extraordinary receipt[6] and what I use a great quantity of and find it very effectuall. If wee continue a farther correspondance (which I shall bee very willing to doe) I desyre he may bee more perticuler in his Invoyce and then shall bee better able to send them to his satisfaction. I have putt up the Cordiall water[7] in large Stone Bottles (accept the Tiracle water[8] the quantity of which being large I have putt in a Rundlett[9]) which I cannott but thinke are better then Keggs which would bee apt to leake out and if a quart or 2

2 Gamboge is a gum resin obtained from *Garcinia hanburii*, a deciduous tree of Cambodia, whence the name. Although valued as a bright yellow dye, gamboge was primarily used as a drastic purgative (Quincy *Complete English Dispensatory* 197; OED; *Ency. Brit.* 11: 439). Eyton's doctor must have been well informed, for gamboge was a rather new drug not mentioned in Salmon's *Pharmacopoeia* of 1716 and first introduced into *Pharmacopoeia Londinensis* in the 1724 edition (E. St John Brooks *Sir Hans Sloane* [London 1954] 84).

3 Millilett is a millet native to India, cultivated as a cereal crop in southern Europe (OED). Salmon valued the ashes of the stalks against struma and a decoction of the seeds to provoke sweat and urine, expel kidney gravel, and cure ague, and a paste applied externally dried up catarrhs in the head or milk in the breasts. Salmon also recommended mixing it with tar and applying this to venomous bites (*Pharmacopoeia* 70, 133).

4 Plague water was a wine or brandy-based remedy, infused with an array of medicinal herbs and roots, valued as an antidote to plague and poisons. This was a type of medicine rather than a specific one, some recipes for which are given in Quincy *Complete English Dispensatory* 366-7.

5 Surfeit water, a medicinal water intended to cure the effects of intemperate eating or drinking, but more widely used against fevers and fits (OED)

6 Recipe

7 Cordial waters are a category of stimulating medicinal drinks valued for digestion, cooling fevers, and as vehicles for other medicines. Cruttenden is probably here referring to the plague and surfeit water. See Salmon *Pharmacopoeia* 395 for an example.

8 Treacle water, the specific kind of plague water sent here, is described by Salmon as containing green walnut juice, rice juice, carduus, marigolds, bawm, butterbur roots, burdock roots, angelica, masterwort, scordium leaves, old Venice treacle, Mithridate, canary wine, white vinegar and lemon juice. It was considered an antidote to plague and poisons, and a cordial in fevers (*Pharmacopoeia* 395-6).

9 Rundlett, or runlet, was a cask of varying size. A 1674 reference cites it as 18½ gallons (OED, s.v. 'runlet').

should wast that way it would bee more then the price of the Bottles which must allsoe bee worth the money there. I have taken great care in the package and hope nothing can suffer any damage, you see by the Invoyce what is conteined in every parcell that he may easyly see as hee opens them, and bee satisfyed thereat. In Concideration you have (as you write) noe partner I have consigned them to you and Mr Thomas Perkins who is a person I have had long dealing with and am well satisfyed with, and therefore I thinke you cannott take it Amisse being soe much a stranger to you that I joyne him with you; But if there bee noe demurr made but the returnes bee made as you promise in your letter by the first man of warr in peices of 8 (unlesse I advice otherwise) I shall bee content to allow you your full Commision as if you hade noe partner in concideration of your securing the Invoyce and I shall satisfy him beside. I shall expect your complyance with what you promise being a great deale of money for me to bee out off and more indeed then I can well afford but being very willing to trade abroad if it may bee to any advantag, I am sure noe one can afford to doe it better; As to the Draw back you mentiond tis soe difficult to gett the persons downe to the Custome house that I found it impossible to gett it done soe gave it over. You will find in one of the cases a small paper parcell directed for Mr Timothy Babington att the George Taverne in Kings Towne as alsoe an inclosed letter soe directed. They are the goods of a perticular* [in margin: Mr Joseph Alleine Writeing Mrs] Friend of mine who desyred they might bee putt up with my things. And his desyre is they may bee delivered to Mr Babington if alive. If he should bee dead the Gentleman desyres you to open them and dispose of them to the best advantage you can and make returns with mine and keepe that account distinct by itself the parcell conteines – A dozen silk printed Hanchercheifs att: 6s 6d A Watch – – – – – att 5 – But the little parcell within directed to Mrs. Babington deliver to her tho he should bee dead. This with hearty service etc.

Postscript I am now come to the 15 day of February; before now I hoped these would have reacht you for the goods have been shipt 2 months but the Fleet have been strangly retarded but are now just hurrying away. I have sent another Invoyce and Bill of Loading inclosed in Mr Perkins Letter.

[in margin: Sent this letter with Invoyce and Bill of Loading in Capt Madden and another Coppy of the same att the same time in Capt Roberts in the Robert and Francis]

19 MR THOMAS PERKINS

Lond Jan: 18 1710/11

SIR

I received yours by Capt Roberts with the 10 hoggsheads of Sugar But I must let you know my resentment of your management in that affayr; the Sugar was bought a great deal to dear being very ordinary. There was a great deale came by the Fleet at 10s a hundred better and 4s or 5s a hundred Cheaper and the price being soe high and the Freight soe extravagantly dear I made a very poor hand of it; I sold the sugars but for 32s 9d a hundred soe that I did not make above 85£ Clear of them soe that I am conciderably a looser of the prime cost of the Invoyce of goods I sent out with you which you know was more then that. If you had sent of the finest sort of Sugar it would have gone off much better and would have cost noe more Freight and Customes but it was soe ordinary that every body blowed[1] upon them. I hade as good very near from Barbados last year that cost above 10 Shillings a hundred lesse and the Freight not much above half as much. You mention in none of your letters what becomes of the remainder of the effects in your hands upon the former account you told me when you came away from Jamaica you hade sold about 40£ worth of the goods but I never heard anything of the money and what you left in Mr Fernlys hands when you came away I never received anything off. I hope you will sett all these matters in a clear light and doe me justice in the case, which I cannot but have an opinion you will doe notwithstanding all these complaints and therefore I now putt another oportunity into your hands of shewing you the respect I bear to you. The case is thus: I sometime agoe received a letter from Mr Richard Eyton (a gentleman I have a small aquaintance with) conteining an Invoyce of Druggs Amounting to: 294£-17s-11d which hee writes word he has agreed with a Gentleman att Jamaica to take off upon their arrivall there, att Cent per Cent advance present money in peices of 8; now my aquaintance with Mr Eyton being but small and he not mentioning the persons name who he hade sold them to and the sume being large I was afrayd to venture it intirely to his management and therefore have joyned you the Bill of Ladeing with him, and will allow you half the Commissions tho if they are disposed of according to his advice and the returnes made by Fleet in concideration hee procured the Invoyce will allow him his whole Commission as if noe other person were concerned in him.

---

1 Blow upon, to defame or discredit (OED, s.v. 'blow')

And therefore I desyre you to satisfye yourself well of the person that is to have them before you deliver them you may discourse Freindly with Mr Eyton (who I have advised I have joyned you with) for I desyre there may bee noe jealousy nor uneasyness between you and I hope there will not. You will sea by the Invoyce the Quantitys are very large and manny of them very valuable goods and wish they may turne to a good account. They are all good and very Cheape and I am a great deal of money out about them. Therefore desyre returnes may bee made by the Fleet, For his positive agreement was to pay presently in Forreigne Silver soe desyre they may bee sent in Man of warr; if I see cause to have any part in any other Comodity shall give you timely advice either by packett boat or some other conveyance. If you send any Sugars in returne of what is yet behind I desyre they may bee the very finest that can bee bought for the Freight and Customes of such is noe more and such I can use in my owne busynesse. I desyre your industrious Application in this affayr for my Advantage who will always remaine   Your Loveing Freind   JC

[*in margin:* Sent this letter with inclosed invoyce and Bill of loading in Capt Roberts: etc and Another Coppy att the same time by Captaine Madden]

20

Jan: 22 1710/11

Wrote to Mr Edward Bulkely[1] att Fort St George in East India By his Nephew Mr Thomas Bulkely And advised him of the receipt of his and that I had received of Madam Fawkner the Balance of his old Accounts to 1708 since which hade sent him 2 parcells amounting to 73-5-½ which advised him his sister would pay the first parcell: 21-8-3 about Lady day and for the remainder hoped to have orders by next ships about it, if not would draw on him next year for the remainder etc.

---

1 Edward Bulkley (d. 1714) had experience in India before being sent out as East India Company Fort Surgeon at Madras in 1692. 'The ingenious Dr. Bulkley' acted as a physician until 1709, thereafter becoming a member of the Madras Council, storekeeper, paymaster, and justice (H.D. Love *Vestiges of Old Madras, 1640-1800* 4 vols. [London, 1913] 1: 563-5; 2: 16-18, 68, 69, 83, 90-2, 103, 145-6). Bulkley contributed many specimens to the herbarium of Charles Dubois; see William Foster *The East India House* (London 1924) 121.

21 TO MR WATERHOUSE FREENLY ATT JAMAICA

Feb: 13 1710/11

SIR

I have not been favoured with any Line from you for above a year; I thinke the last I received from you mentioned you hade disposed of those cases of Waters master Perkins hade left with you but I heare nothing of any returnes you have made and hope you have not for if you have it is lost. I hope you will by the next good Conveyance Ballance that small matter. Allsoe should bee glad to heare whether you have done any thing with Spaine who I heare is in good Circumstances enough to pay if he will; what hee writes of ordering one to pay it here is a meer sham for I have writt to the person and he disownes he has any effects of his in his hands and therefore I desyre you will presse him and threaten him if hee will not comply without; I never tooke a farthing of him in my life and tis very hard I should loose all. Allsoe in your letter you mentioned that Smithwick being dead that mony was all lost But that Capt Vassall hade generously promised to pay the first cost which I have writ to him about by this Conveyance but know not how to direct to him perticulerly but hope it will come to him to give him thanks for his kind offer   Yours

Advised him if he made any returnes in Sugar to let it bee of the finest sort etc.

[*in margin:* Sent by Capt Roberts]

22 TO CAPT SAMUELL VASSALL ATT JAMAICA

Feb 13 1710/11

WORTHY SIR

By a letter I sometime since received from Mr Fernly I understand that Smithwick is dead who owed the money to my Cousin John Viner and that there was noe prospect of receiveing any part of it; I am sorry it was not followed while hee lived if it had I understand it might have been received but now is to late. However I cannot but thankfully owne your great favour in giveing timely notice of it and perticulerly for your generous offer which hee advices me you have made freely to allow me what I am out of pockett on

that Account. As I formerly hinted to you Mr Shepherd to whom Mr John
Viner was indebted prest very hard upon him for the money and threatned
hee would ruine his Credit if hee did not pay him; about the time he came to
you this hapned, when my Cosin viner wrote to me to endeavour to bring Mr
Shepard to a temper and this I endeavoured what I could but could worke
him to nothing, he was absolutely resolved he would blow him up, those were
his words. When I found I could doe nothing else with him I asked him what
he would take for his debt not intending in the least to buy it att first; but he
demanding much lower then I expected I tooke him att his word haveing allwayes found Cozen John Viner just to me in greater Concernes; what I actually gave him was 10 Guineys but the obtaineing the proof of the debt befor
the Lord Major, the letters of Attourney and other charges amount it to
about 12 pounds which if you are soe kind as to pay I shall owne as a signall
favour and what I could never have expected if you hade not generously
offered it. I leave the Method of doing it wholly to yourself whether by goods,
Bill or Forreigne Silver by man of warr; I know you are better aquainted
with these matters then I and doe not question but after you have made soe
kind an offer you will doe it in a way most to my advantage   Remaine etc.

[*in margin:* Sent by Capt Roberts]

23 MR THOMAS BARTON

London: March 3: 1710/11

SIR

Yours of Nov. 21 1710 by her Majestys Shipp Norwich and New Hampshire
came both safe to hand with 100 ozs peices of 8/8 for whiche returne you
hearty thankes as allsoe with Invoyce of a parcell of wares which have shipt
you by this Conveyance viz Capt Tayler in the Unity. Inclosed is bill of
Loading and Invoyce of the sayd parcell which wish well and safe to your
hands and to your Content which I have endeavoured and every thing sent
are of the best and charged very low. All are sent accept the Liquid Snush,[1]

---

1 A liquid snuff is described by Quincy as the juice obtained by pressing the leaves of honeysuckle,
betony, primrose, and marjoram. This was either snuffed from the hand or blown up the nose
with a quill. It was used to clear the nose and, unlike solid snuff, did not itself clog the nose
(*Complete English Dispensatory* 687).

the Spiritt of Scurvy grasse,[2] and Stoughtons Elixir[3] which the time being soe
short could not well procure; but you may expect them by the next shipps
which are allready putt [up?] and hope will Sayle in a Month att farthest,
shall allsoe then send you Bottles or att least write fully to you about that
matter these shipps hurrying away faster then was expected have no time to
write soe fully as intended but shall by the next. I observe by your Account
Sent you charge me Debtor for Freight £1 18s by which I know not what you
meane being a new thing I never heard of before and what noe person I ever
delt with ever desyred and therefore can by noe meanes allow of. Which I
thinke your letter fully answeares, for you write returnes by bills of Exchange
are 60 perCent and if You advance but 75£ on the goods then there remaines
but 15 perCent which sure is not an Equivalent for the Hazzard of the Sea
where losses must be expectd unlesse insurance bee made which will amount
to more the[n] profitt. Therefore tho I am very willing to trade with and
would give you all incouragement possible yet if I should tell you I am willing
to deale soe as to loose by it I dare say you will not beleive me nor there is noe
reason you should. Allsoe In that account suppose you omitt the Elixir
Salutis[4] and Aqua Hungaria[5] which you formerly disputed for tho you had

2 *Cochlearia*, a grass common in Scotland and parts of England, was reputed to prevent scurvy on
long sea voyages. The juice was considered useful for liver and spleen swellings, and for healing
mouth and skin sores and ulcers. See *ibid.* 325; Culpeper *English Physician* 343; Salmon
Pharmacopoeia 42; Grieve *Modern Herbal* 2: 725.

3 A year later Richard Stoughton received a patent for ' "a new and most usefull restorative cordial and medicine" known by the name of "Stoughton's elixir magnum stomachicu" or "the
great cordial elixir" otherwise called "the stomatick tincture or bitter drops" ' (Great Britain,
Patent Office *Abridgments of Specifications Relating to Medicine, Surgery, and Dentistry ... A.D. 1620-1866*
2nd ed. [London 1872] 2). Stoughton's elixir would be very popular in eighteenth-century America, and it is interesting that this nostrum was known before it was patented in England (James
Young and G.B. Griffenhagen 'Old English Patent Medicines in America' *Chemist and Druggist*
167 (1957); 716). Its continuing popularity in England, at 1 shilling a bottle in 1748, is shown by
its inclusion in Poplicola 'Pharmacopoeia Empirica, or the List of Nostrums and Empirics' *The
Gentleman's Magazine* 18 (1748): 348.

4 Invented by an English clergyman in the mid-seventeenth century, Duffy's *elixir salutis* became so
popular in the eighteenth century, and so well known, that its complete formula was printed, not
only in Robert James's *Medicinal Dictionary, with a History of Drugs* 3 vols. (London 1743-5) but
eventually in John Wesley's *Primitive Physic* 23rd ed. (London 1791) (reprinted London 1960)
121. Senna leaves, gueiacum chips, elecampane root, aniseed, caraway, coriander, liquorice, and
raisins were steeped in French brandy, the solids removed, and the liquor drunk as a purgative
and carminative. This nostrum, the first to be advertised in an American newspaper, was recommended to readers of the *Boston Newsletter* as early as 4 October 1708; see Young and Griffenhagen 'Old English Patent Medicines' 716. Also see Poplicola 'Pharmocopoeia Empirica' 348.
S. Stander notes, 'It was used in the treatment of infant disorders and probably did much to increase mortality,' 'Transatlantic Trade in Pharmaceuticals during the Industrial Revolution'
Bull. Hist. of Med 43 [1969]: 339).

5 See above, letter 13, note 1.

not then disposed of them yet hope you have by this time or att least will and make me returnes: and as to those ways you mention of makeing returnes shall advice about it and give you my thoughts by the next ships remaine att present   Yours   JC

[*in margin:* This letter sent by Capt Tayler And another Coppy by Capt Holberton]

2 4

Aprill 13: 1711

I wrote largely to you by Capt Holberton and Capt Tayler by the latter shipt you good[*s*]; this comes to advice you have put up your Liquid Snush, Spirit of Scurvygrasse, and Stomach Tincture[1] in a Box which I have putt up with Mr Savages goods. I was afraid the Box being small might mis carry alone. Inclosed is Invoyce of the same. I cannot possitively assert the Tincture to bee the same with Stoughtons but it is very near it and I beleive as good; I gott all the light I could possible into his Medicine and I dare affirme this will per- forme whatever his will; you may give them the same directions about take- ing them. Your Shipps hurrying away in such hast (tho they stay long enough after they are gone to the Westward for the whole fleet is still att Portsmouth) that I hade not oppertunity to put up your Cask of ½ pint Bottles but by the first good opertunity shall doe it. I cannot tell what to say about the returnes you mention in fish by way of Lysbon. It [*blot:* is?] what I doe not understand and therefore had much rather have it as formerly in Silver or in good Bills of Exchange or if Turpentine [*in margin:* bee cheap and the Freight low you may send some of it if you can't gett Silver; shall Adde noe more etc.]

25 MR HABIJAH SAVAGE

London March: 3: 1710/11

SIR

Your 3 letters of Nov. 13 last came all safe to hand with the 160 ozs peices of 8/8 per her Majesty's Ship Norwich for which give you hearty thankes. All- soe received your inclosed Invoyce for another parcell of wares which I have complyed and Shipt on board the Unity Capt Tayler Invoyce and Bill of

1 Stoughton's elixir

Loading of which parcell comes inclosed Which wish well to your hand and to your satisfaction. These Shipps hurrying away very quickly after the arrivall of your Fleet there are some few things omitted of which you see an account att the foot of your Invoyce; which things you may expect by the next shipps that sayle which hope will bee in a month att farthest they being allready putt up and a good part of their loading ready which these shipps could not take in. You will observe inclosed Bill of Ladeing and Invoyce and Bill of Loading of a Chest or Case Conteining a cwt of Dryed Liquorish and shipt you last year in the Nicholson Capt Partis which Ship was unhappyly taken by the French when she was allmost arrived att New England but was afterward retaken by a Dutch Privateer and brought in here. Severall parcells of her Cargoe were plundered in the time the French hade her in possession, there is not a certaine Account what goods remaine but by what account there is yours is left; soe hope by the next ships allsoe to send it which was the reason I did not putt up any dry Liquorish new because I hope to send that. A perticuler account of all that matter expect by next oppertunity. I heartily wish these things safe to your hands and to your full Contentment they being the best of every sort and very well Bought   remaine Sir Yours   JC

[*in margin:* This letter sent by Capt Tayler and Another Coppy by Capt Holberton]

26 [*Habijah Savage*]

London Aprill 5. 1711

SIR

I am now arrived to Aprill 5 1711. Above is Coppy of what writt you by sundry conveyances and this serves to inclose Invoyce and Bill of Loading of the remaineing part of former Invoyce omitted before for the reasons there mentioned which I have shipt you in the Swann Friggat Capt John Buckler which wish well to your hands and every way to your content. You will find in the case no i A Box mark't T B: which I desyre you will please to deliver upon demand to Mr Thomas Barton. I have advised him of it that I have Shipt it in your Case the reason was the Box was soe small that I was afraid it would miscarry if sent alone; he will pay his proportion of Freight for it. Every thing in your first order is now sent acccpt onely the Prunes which are not to be hade, sorry stuff good for nothing have been sold for 7s a pound and allsoe the Bezoar oriental is omitted being att such an extravagant price that it discouraged me from sending of any. I cannot yet give you soe good an account of the case of Liquorish which was taken but I am assured it is remaining but the owners of the Ship are not come to a resolve whether she shall take in her goods againe and proceed her voyage or let the goods bee shipt on some other Shipp. I hope I shall bee able to give you a full account by the Mast shipps, you may I thinke depend upon receiveing it one way or other ere it be long. When that Case arrives you will find in it a small Box directed For Mr Thomas Greaves att Charles Town which I have advised him of and desyre you will please to deliver to him he paying his proportion of Freight. Wee have in expectation of some ships from New England a great while but they are not yet arrived. As to returnes I cannott tell how to give other directions then formerly vizt in Silver if possible to bee had or in good bills of exchange, all Comoditys are very low. There is a New Tax layd upon dear Skins and all Furrs of 12d in the pound.[1] Whatever goods you send pray let them bee the best of the kind; Turpentine or oyl if bought Cheape may doe pretty well but after all if it bee to bee hade I hade much rather have Silver   Yours   JC

27 MR WILLIAM LITTLE OF BOSTON

London Mar: 5: 1710/11

SIR

The above is Coppy of what I writt you by Capt Partis last year with your goods And this comes to advice you that that Ship was unhappyly taken by the French when she was gott allmost to New England and in some time after was retaken by the Dutch and brought in here. But tho She has been in here above 2 Months yet I cannot gett a perfect account of what goods remaine on board her (for the French plundered her of a good part of her Cargoe while she was in their possession) but by the best account I can meet with yet I find your Trunk has escaped them which I hope will prove true. The place the Ship is brought into is the farthest part of England near 300 miles from London but when the matter is settled and every Freighter has prooved his interest and payd the Salvage (which to bee sure will bee large) wee hope the goods will either bee shipt againe on the same Ship and she proceed her voy-

---

1 There were increases in the customs on skins and furs in 1711, by 9 Anne c 11, and again the following year, though these had not even reached the discussion stage in the Commons when Cruttenden wrote this letter. See L.E. Stock, *Proceedings and Debates of the British Parliaments respecting North America* 5 vols. (Washington 1924-41) 3: 294-5. Rates varied for different skins and furs, but the impositions of both years on deer skin constituted increased duties of 10d per pound.

age againe, or else some other Ship will call for them and take them on board as they goe by which way ever it bee I shall take all the care I can in your Interest and doe for you as other Freighters doe for their Freinds; I am very sorry for this misfortune but tis often the fate of Merchant Adventurers. I hade a Chest on board of my owne that suffered the same fate and I shall act just for you as I doe for my self and advice you by these next Shipps what stepps I have made in the affayr. I hope att last the things will come safe to your hands tho there will bee charges upon them which would not have been if this accident hade not hapned.

28 TO MR GEORGE JACKSON[1] OF PISCATAQUA IN NEW ENGLAND

Mar: 5: 1710/11

SIR

I received yours from Barbados with account you were designeing for New England with your Invoyce for Druggs and Medicines which you desyred might bee forwarded by Capt Sherburn which I designed but poor Gentleman he hade the Misfortune to have his Ship burnt here soon after she was put up. I allsoe received yours of Nov. 23 from Piscattaqua rejoyce to heare you are gott safe to New England. Your Invoyce I have complyed with and designe to Ship them by the very next ships that sayle which will bee within a Month att most; I thought to have Shipt them on Capt Tayler but could not gett Freight but shall not fayle you by the next. Desyre you to make what expedition you can in disposeing of those things you allready have that soe returnes may bee made by the next masst Fleet; I thought fitt to give you this advice that you may be satisfyed of the reason why you hade not the goods by these first Shipps but that you may depend on them by the next the danger of the seas excepted   Yours etc

29

SIR

I am now arrived to the 18 of Aprill the above is coppy of what I writt you per last shipps which hope you have received. This serves farther to advice

1 George Jackson, a surgeon of Marblehead, Mass., served in this capacity to the Phips expedition to Quebec in 1690. In 1702 he bought a farm at Scituate, later moving to Piscataqua (Farmer *Genealogical Register* 159; Savage *Genealogical Dictionary* 2: 529; Ernest Myrand *1690: Sir William Phips Devant Québec* [Quebec 1893] 217). Jackson's account for medicines for the expedition is in *ibid.*, 295-6. Also see Byron Fairchild's study of Jackson's in-laws, *Messrs William Pepperrell* 107.

you that I have shipt your Invoyce of Druggs and Medicines on board the Swan Friggat Capt Buckler Invoyce and bill of Loading of which comes inclosed. Wish them well to your hand and to your contentment and a good markett. There are not above 3 or 4 things omitted some I could not tell what you ment by them; the Sal viperarid[1] you writ for 8 ozs I suppose you did not concider the price, it would have cost me 16£. The lowest farthing I ever bought it for in life was 40s an ounce I suppose you would bee loath to give soe much with advance; if you are willing to give soe there is a freind of mine one Mr Thomas Greaves of Charles Towne who writ to me for an ounce about 2 yeares agoe which I sent him and when it came the price frighted him and he has sent to me to take it againe. He will bee glad to part with it to you; you may make the best termes with him you can for it. Allsoe you writ for large quantitys of severall Chymicall oyles as Lavender and Mint which rise high, being deare I have sent some of each but not as much as you writt for. I have charged your Invoyce as low as I sell them to any here for ready money and therefore the proposall I make with you is either for you to pay for them here in ready money and you run the risque of the seas or, in goods which I shall dispose of to the best advantage I can and give you credit for the Ballance; or else with 75£ perCent advance upon them with you in your money and I run the risque which is the same foot I deal with all my Chapmen in New England upon. For the most part I have my returnes in peices of 8/8 silver att 8s per ounce[2] which I like better then any other and which they allways send by the man of Warr put up in a Bagg and sealed and take 3 Bills of Loading for them to send by other Ships; the Freight is 50s perCent. I desyre you will not fayl of making returnes by the next mast Fleet and shall be glad to settle a Correspondance with you; from me you shall allways have Candid and honest dealing and I promise my self the same from you and hope shall not bee disapoynted. If you send your Comoditys Turpentine or oyle etc I will dispose of them to the best advantage I can but they are all low and there will bee great losse upon them and therefore I really beleive money will bee the best or good bills of Exchange which if you send you must send 3 setts by severall Shipps. Shall adde noe more but remaine   Yours   JC

[*in margin*: As to what you mentioned of sending the Electuary[3] unmixt tis what cannott bee done there beeing gums and other things that cannot bee powdered in them tis such a proposall as I never heard of my life:]

1 *Sal viperarum*
2 This was precisely the Boston price of an ounce of silver that year; see above, p. xix, note 48.
3 Electuary, a type of medicinal paste in which powders and other ingredients are mixed with honey, jams, or syrups (OED).

30 TO MR THOMAS LITTLE ATT PLYMOUTH IN NEW ENGLAND

Mar: 5: 1710[/11]

SIR

I have not been favoured with any letter from you this 2 yeares, I was in hopes of hearing from you last year and this yeare but were both times disapoynted. I hope if you have noe farther occasion or inclination to deale with me you will cleare your old account; you have by former letters hade the ballance sent you which is 50£ 8s 5½d I desyre you will not put me to the uneasye task of writeing again about which is what I am very unwilling to but must have regard to my owne interest; I should have been glad of a farther Correspondance with you but if are other ways engaged I wish you one that may please you better and remaine   Yours etc.   JC

31 TO MR CONRADE ADAMS ATT BARBADOS

Aprill 3 1712 –

SIR

I received Severall letters from you last year by the fleet and allsoe the inclosed Invoyce from Mr William Phyllips which have complyed with and shipt in Capt Potts invoyce and Bill of Loading of which comes inclosed; I wish them well to your hands and to Mr Phyllips intyre satisfaction. I hope I may intirely depend on your promise of makeing full remittances by next good opertunity for it was a conciderable disapoyntment not to have them last year haveing (as I hinted to you in my last letters) hade an occasion since of shipping me of all the money I could gett togather. I observe your complaints of the Dearnesse of the things sent you but cannot see ground for it; everything out of my way was bought with ready money or very small creditt and as hard as I could and what was in my owne way was as cheap as I sell them to any of my owne trade here and I am sure the advance upon them will scarce make good the losse upon returnes in case the effects come safe. Hope there will bee noe complaints about these things or any other for the future for I doe not love to have them. I hope you will still use your endeavours for procureing what Invoyces you can which I shall allways bee ready to comply with. I am sorry you are like to gett noe more of Dr Houghs debt; I cannot but thinke there was a neglect there for if you hade got security beforc his circumstances were soe bade it might have been recovered. Tis a great deale of money to loose and more then I feare I shall ever make up by any tradeing to your Island and Therefore I hope you will account yourself under some kind of obligation to endeavour to promote my interest what you can in order to reimburse me what I have lost. If the effect bee not sent by the spring Fleet I desyre you will ship them one half in Capt Potts and the other in some good Shipp: and give me as timely notice as possible either by way of Bristoll or any other way you can that I may make insurance. I have often writt to you and desyre now againe that if you can possible I may have a hoggshead or 2 of first white Sugars which would bee fitt for my owne occasions and save me buying it elsewhere; allsoe if you can meet with any Aloes would bee glad of some not exceeding a 1000 lbs weight. I leave the matter to your management to act as much for my Interest as you can which I doe not question but you will. You will observe inclosed is a letter directed to you from Major Johnson who is my uncle by whom I understand that you have about 300£ of his effects in your hands which hee has desyred you to ship by the next fleet; now I request the favour of you that when ever you send his effects you would not fayle of giveing me an account of it by what ship in what goods and what quantity that I may have advice of it as soon or before he can have it. The reason of my request is this: I have a sister which lives with him a widdow and hee has a 1000£ of hers in his hands all she has for herself and Child and hee has faithfully promised her she shall have that money as part of her debt but, hee haveing broke his word with her in the like case severall times, wee are willing if possible to secure this; for in short his circumstances are growne very low and wee are afraid she will loose her money and would bee glad if possible to secure some part of it att leaste. Keepe this to yourself. Inclosed is a letter to Mr Phyllips which please to deliver with the Chest. This is the needful etc.

[*in margin*: Sent by the Mary, Capt Winter and Another by the Barbados Merchant, Capt Plumsted and Another by the Susannah and Hannah, Capt Potts.]

32 FOR MR WILLIAM PHYLLIPS ATT BARBADOS

Apr: 3 1712

SIR

I was favoured with yours under Covert of Mr Conrade Adams with your small Invoyce which I have put up and sent by this Conveyance in Capt Richard Potts which I wish well to your hand and to your content and full satisfaction which I have endeavoured, everything being of the best and the prizes very low. I thought myself bound to let you know how much I value you and your Custome and to assure you I shall allways bee ambitious to serve you and whatever Invoyces I receive from you or your Freinds shall all-ways bee complyed with and forwarded by the first opertunity. This is the needfull att present but hearty service etc from   JC

[*in margin*: Sent 2 coppys inclosed in Mr Adamss']

33 MR GEORGE GREEMES ATT BARBADOS

London Apr: 7 1712

I take this opertunity to aquaint you that I have received the full Ballance of your account by your good Friend Mr Roylee and allsoe to returne you my hearty thankes for your care in that affayr and to assure you that I shall att all times bee ambitious to serve you or any Freind of yours and shall take care to doe it in such a way as may proove to your advantage and shall prevent for the future any such ill consequences as happened by not sending the Bill of Loading by the same ship the goods were sent; but it was an uncomon case and wherein many more and for farr greater concernes then mine were in the case, the ship sayleing before any one expected it. This I thought my self obliged to informe you which is the needfull att present from Sir Yours   JC

[*in margin*: Sent in the Barbados Merchant, Capt Plumsted And another in the Elizabeth, Capt Chandler]

34 TO MR HABIJAH SAVAGE ATT BOSTON IN NEW ENGLAND

Apr [4?] 1712

SIR

I was favoured with yours with inclosed Invoyce as allsoe that by her majestys ship Adventure wherein you have given me an account you have shipt 25 Barrells of oyle in Capt Savage. I have put of[f] writeing till this day in hopes of the fleet arriveing which have been lookt for this 2 months but not yet come, onely one to Bristoll which parted from the fleet soon after they came and Capt Holberton who was taken by the French and retaken againe by one of our men of warr, soe that wee are like to have a very bad account of the rest, God knows when wee shall hear of them. I have made noe insurance partly for want[1] of money and partly because the Ensurers want insureing. I ensured upon a ship that was lost above 6 months agoe and cannot gett my money yet soe that here is nothing but discouragements upon trade and noe prospect of a peace soe that I don't see tis worth anyones while to send his effects abroad as things are att present. Yet that I might not disapoynt you I have complyed with your Invoyce exept a few things which shall send by the next Ship and have forwarded them to you by the Prince Eugene which I wish well to you and to your content. The dry things are all putt up by themselves and the other by themselves soe that it is impossible anything can come to any Damage without extraordinary carelessenesse. You have inclosed a Bill of Loading and invoyce of these goods now sent and allsoe a small paper wherein it hinted what is not sent att all or what in a lesse Quantity then you ordered. The Liquorish have not sent because I expecte the 100 weight of that which I formerly sent and which was taken will come to you as soon as this arrives; I have paid one half the value of it againe for Salvage and is now with the rest of the goods in that Ship put on board another ship bound for New England soe hope it will come to you att last. The Saffron[2] I sent none because of the extreame dearnesse of it; I cannot buy it heare under 4 pound 10s per lb and for the Spiritts of Scurvygrasse the time of yeare is not farr enough advanced for them; but there [is] another ship putt up, the Portugall Gally which will sayle in about a Months time by whom I hope to send what remaines of your Invoyce. I live in hopes shall have some news of the Masst fleet before these ships are quite gone and hope shall have some farther returnes from you besides the oyl which you have advised off or else it will bee a very great disapoyntment to me haveing etc. The goods sent you are all very good and bought as low as possible being willing to give you all manner of incouragement: that if possible may continue a correspondance togather. The Rad Turpeth[3] is not to bee hade nor you must not expect it; there has

---

1 'What' in MS

2 The dried stigma and part of the style of the autumnal saffron crocus, used as an edible yellow food dye, was highly regarded as in ingredient in cordials. Salmon regarded saffron as the greatest of all vegetable cordials – tonic, poison resister, cure for plague, fevers, obstructions, asthma, etc., and prolonging life and health (*Pharmacopoeia* 108). Thomas Thacher had, in 1688, recommended saffron over the butter cordials for relief of smallpox victims in Boston. His broadside suggested saffron in milk on the fourth day of the disease, and saffron in malaga wine later (reprinted in Gordon *Aesulapius Comes to the Colonies* 112-13). See also *Ency. Brit.* 23:999; OED; Grieve *Modern Herbal* 2:698-700.

3 *Rad turpethi*, known also as Kirshna turpeth or deadly carrot, is a powerful purgative from the root of the East Indian jallop. In 1716 Salmon valued it as an 'eminent' purger of 'gross and clammy Humours,' while indicating that it caused nausea and vomiting if taken alone and was dangerous for children or pregnant women (*Pharmacopoeia* 17). By 1736 Quincy reported that it was no longer used (*Complete English Dispensatory* 202). Also see OED; Grieve *Modern Herbal* 2:823.

been none for many yeares; wee use Jallep[4] for it hear which serves as well. The browne paper is all sent but 15 Quire; There is of 3 sorts of it which I thought was better than to send it all of one sort you may see which sorts are alike by laying them togather, I saved you half apeice in the paper for there is a very large duty layd upon it But I bought it just before the Tax commenced and soe saved you that money.[5] Allsoe the Lapis Bezoard[6] is extravagantly Dear; it cost me 4£ an ounce every farthing and soe has all that I have used myself for a year and half past;I beleive I shall send noe more of that yett. Hope to have opertunity of writeing againe before these ships are quite gone, shall adde noe more now but etc.

[*in margin*: Coppys sent in the Sarah Gally, Capt Achison and by the Prince Eugene, Capt Wakefeild and by the Portugall Gally, Capt Morris]

35

[*14 May 1712*]

SIR

I am now arrived to May 14 and take this opertunity by Capt Morris in the Portugall Gally to informe you that the Mast Fleet are arrived 3 weekes agoe in Ireland where they still remaine and how much longer they may lye there I know not. The Caswell Friggott is arrived among them but feare her lying soe long there will be a detriment to her oyle; the cask will if not very good leak in hott weather. I have spoke severall times with Mr Blettsoe who is my perticuler Freind and hee promises to pay me the 100£ Sterling when hee receives the Bill of the Government but there is noe prospect of that this year. They have not yet soe much as accepted the Bill; all the Bills drawne on the Government on the Expedition are in the same case as I doubt not you have been sufficiently satisfyed off: I mention this to let you know I am in noe expectation of receiveing that this 8 or 9 Months[1] and therefore hope you will provide accordingly some other way. I shall God willing send what remaines

4 Jalap, root of *Convolvulus jalapa*, a South American and Mexican bindweed valued as a strong purgative. Like turpeth, jalap was powerful enough to cause griping, a characteristic which in both cases was to be offset by adding liquorice, cloves, cinnamon or ginger (Salmon *Pharmacopoeia* 10; Quincy *Complete English Dispensatory* 201; OED).

5 By 9 Anne c. 11 substantial duties were imposed upon vellum and parchment as of 24 June 1711 (*Statutes* 12:144).

6 Bezoar stones

1 The redemption of bills resulting from the Walker expedition to Quebec were still under discussion in the House of Commons in June of 1717 (Stock *Proceedings and Debates* 3: 390-1).

of former Invoyce with the additions in your letter by the next ship which will sayle in a month or thereabouts and shall then advice if anything farther materiall present about the Bill or any other thing occurr nessessaryly, which is the needfull att present etc.

36 TO MR WILLIAM LITTLE ATT BOSTON

Apr: 15 1712

SIR

This comes to informe you what steps I have taken in your unhappy affayr: I have by severall conveyances advised you that the ship Nicholson wherein I shipt your Bookes etc was taken and retaken againe and brought into Plymouth and that I hoped they would have been shipt againe long ere now but there has been unaccountable Remoras[1] in the way for tho tis 14 months since the Ship was brought in yet the Captors being Dutch and the Freighters could not or would not agree about the salvage soe that it has hung in suspence ever since and a great many of the goods are quite spoyled besides those plundered att first. But att last they are agreed upon one half Salvage according to the Appraisement [*in margin*: 6£ 17s 6d valued att.] accordingly I have paid the one half of their appraisement which was 3£ 8s 9d and for charges of warehouse roome att the rate of 6 per cent 8s and there is a ship now gone downe to take them in and I hope att last they will reach you. I am very sorry you should meet with such disapoyntments but it was noe fault of mine; I have acted all along in the matter as if the case were my owne; I hope to write againe when I hear the goods are shipt. In the meantime remaine etc.
                                                                          JC

[*in margin*: Sent inclosed in Mr Savages letter in Capt Achison]

37 TO MR THOMAS BARTON

May 14 1712

SIR

This serves to informe you I have received your 3 letters by the Mast Fleet and your Invoyce therein and observe the Contents; But the ship this comes by being just ready to sayle have not time to answeare the perticulers but

---

1 Remoras are a sucking fish supposed to slow the ship to which they were attached; obstruction, impediment (OED). Also known as 'suck-stone' or 'stop-ship' (Josselyn *New England's Rarities* 29).

cheifly send this to advice you I shall send your Invoyce by the next shipp that will sayle in a Month or 6 weekes time and shall then write att large and take notice of the manny perticulers of your letter and allsoe send this that you may have a dependance on receiving your orders, the danger of the Seas only accepted. Hope you will forward your remittances by the next good opertunity haveing been much disapoynted for want of them this conveyance. Shall observe your orders punctually in everything and remaine etc.   JC

38 TO MR THOMAS LITTLE

May: 14 1712

SIR

I am favoured with yours per the Mast Fleet and heartyly begg pardon if there were any thing in my last to you that gave offence I am sure I did not designe it for that end. I allsoe received yours last sumer with the Bill of 20£ on Mr Love which was punctually paid for which I returne you hearty thankes and have given your account Creditt for it. What remaines farther in your hands which according to my account is 30£ 8s 5½d you mention you had returned by this Fleet if I hade given orders in what it should bee in. I thinke I ever since I hade any dealings with you left it to you to make returnes in what you thought best; I hade rather have it if it can bee procured in Silver Money by man of Warr or in Bills of Exchange but if you can gett neither, Turpentine is the best Comodity now; how long it may keepe soe I know not but att present it beares a great price or oyle of Turpentine. I have hade it formerly it would doe well now: I take notice that you mention it is 40£ remains in your hands but suppose you mean New England money which brings it to much the same as my 30£ Sterling. I must leave it to your Management to send the Ballance whatever you make it; I doubt not in the least of your doing me justice and therefore willingly aquiesse in you. I received allsoe a letter from your Brother wherein he writes hee designes to come hither this Sumer and for that reason I doe not write to him supposing him come away, if hee persist in that resolution, before a letter could reach him. If hee be not come I desyre you to tell him I shall observe his orders and doe as hee directed in his letter. I know not whether you have left following of Pharmacy, if not and you please to begin a farther Correspondance I promise you shall meet with all the Candour and fayrnesse you can expect. Remaine Yours   JC

[*in margin*: Sent by Capt Morris in the Portugall Gally Aug 25 1712 sent another Coppy in Capt Savage]

39 TO MR GEORGE JACKSON ATT PISCATAQUA NEW ENGLAND

May 14 1712

SIR

Yours I received dated Feb 8 last per the Mast fleet I am glad to heare you received the Medicines safe in Capt Buckler and allsoe that you have recovered your health. I should have been glad of some returnes from you by the mast fleet but understand by yours the reasons why I hade not, I hope and expect you will not fayle me by next returne. I understand you designe to send Beaverstones;[1] now I must advice you that it is but a dull Comodity and if not well cured will wast extreamely in weight and it is very cheap here and therefore unlesse it bee very good and cheape it will not bee worth sending, it is not worth above 5s a pound here and it pays a very large duty; Bills of Exchange or silver money I beleive will doe much better. I thought it nessessary to give you this caution. If you see Mr Emerson give my service to him and let him know I received his letter and shall answeare it by the Mast Fleet by which possibly I may write to you again. Shall bee glad of a further correspondance with you who am etc. Yours   JC

[*in margin*: Sent by Capt Morris in Portugall Gally]

40

July 22 1712

I wrote to him againe by Mr Thomas Drumond Surgeon of the New Hamshire Mast Ship and advised him of the great tax layd upon Castor[1] and allsoc if he sent any of it to send it by Mr Drumond; prest him earnestly to remitt the whole Ballance by next returne of the Mast Fleet. Inclosed in his writt to Mr Emerson advised him rather to send Turpentine Then Castor etc. Note: Wrote to him againe By the Caswell Friggott, Arthur Savage: copy of the former and inclosed another to Mr Emerson.

---

1 Beaverstones are two small glands from the groin of the beaver. They contain a reddish-brown unctuous substance called 'castor' or 'castoreum,' valued in medicine and perfumery (OED, s.v. 'beaver,' 'castor'). Salmon considered beaverstones as having a 'wonderful force' against a wide variety of difficulties, nervous and digestive, and included curing deafness and toothache (*Pharmacopoeia* 183-4).

1 Beaverstones

41 MR HABIJAH SAVAGE

London July 24 1712

SIR

Have wrote largely to you by severall last ships to which referr you; this serves onely to inclose Invoyce and bill of Loading of a small Cargo sent in Capt Cary part of your latter Invoyce, the remainder am prepareing to ship in your Brother which will sayle (as he assures me) att the same time by whom shall write againe and more att large. I have received yours by Capt Kent with a farther Invoyce but observe there are many things in that which are in your former additionall Invoyce soe am ready to conclude you doe not keepe a coppy of it by you. I shall act as prudently as I can in that affayr shall referr all to next oppertunity   Yours   JC

[*in margin*: per Capt Cary]

42 [*Mr Habijah Savage*]

London Aug 25th 1712

SIR

I am now arrived to the 25th of August and this serves to cover Invoyce and Bill of Loading of the residue of your order (not shipt before) Shipt in your Brother Savages ship: which wish well to your hands and to your full Content. I observed before that there [*were*] manny things and the same Quantitys repeated in 2 or 3 of your Invoyces and therefore was att a losse how to manage that affayr: but have done the best I can. What I have set before in the last parcells have omitted here as you will see att one view by the inclosed paper. I have advised you allready about the Bill on the Government what steps have been taken and with how little successe; that affayr remaines still as it was noe part of it received nor noe prospect of it. Your Brother will bee able to informe you about it when you see him; I mention this againe to sett you right that you may not reckon that 100£ as paid soe hope you will regulate yourself with respect to returnes accordingly; intreat you would bee as large as possible by next Mast Fleet. Wee are now in dayly expectation of a peace soe hope trade will not bee soe precarious as formerly. Every thing here is very dull; your oyl I have still by me; cannot sell it for above 21£ per Ton and leave you to judge then of the losse. As to next returnes, if it cannot bee gott in good bills of Exchange or in Silver money I desyre you may send it in Turpentine if not dear and the Freight not to high which hope will now bee more reasonable. If you can buy it that it will come out here about 14 or 15s a hundred you may send me a hundred Barrells if you thinke fitt; it was the best Comodity that came home last year; what it may bee next I know not. I suppose now there will bee ships running often whereby wee may have advice more frequently then formerly. I have hade the misfortune to send a parcell of Druggs by Invoyce to a person in Jamaica who happened to bee dead before they came there, and therefore designe to order my correspondant there to Ship them for you, they being all fresh and good and most of them things in your Invoyce, for which reason have sent somewhat lesse of some things supposing they will serve till the others come. You will observe there is 2 lbs of Spicknard charged in your Bill which is not send the reason is this: I have ordered Mr Thomas Barton to deliver you 2 pound of it he haveing 6 lbs of it by him which I sent him a little while agoe according to his order but he says tis threw a mistake hee designeing it for oyl of Spikenard and he proposes to returne it againe; I have writ to him to deliver 2 lbs to you but if he should not or if hee have desposed of it any other way I shall crosse it out. I charge it att 18s a pound tho if I hade it heare could sell it for 24s a pound there being none in London to bee gott; it cost me 18s a pound when I bought it but when I sent it him it was growne Cheaper soe I charged him[1] but 12s a pound for it. I have sent noe oyl of Spike[*nard*] because I find there is noe such thing truely prepared; tis onely oyl of Turpentine and a little Lavender Spike thrown into the distillation to sweare by[2] (and sometimes not that neither) but the comon oyl of Turpentine is as good and that you have more plenty than wee have. Wee were here in great hopes of Druggs growing cheaper but our wise Parliament have taken care to lay a Tax of 20 perCent on all Druggs soe that instead of falling they are like to bee much dearer. I have inclosed a memorandum of the Druggs I designe to order you from Jamaica if there bee more of any sort then you need you may offer Mr Thomas Barton what quantity he pleases of them they are a choice parcell of fresh goods. I have with this parcell sent your 4 Grosse of Gally potts[3] which I find charged to your last Invoyce tho they were not then sent and therefore have not charged them now I have sent them. You will observe inclosed a bill of loading of the Case with the 1 cwt of dry Liquorish which was shipt you againe in Capt

---

1 [*in margin*: Vide 3 leaves forward] There, the rest of the letter, pp. 95 7 of the manuscript, is given as added here. The addition is headed 'Mr Savages Letter continued from 3 leaves Backward.'

2 Spikenard is now an obsolete name for English lavender (OED), but this latter was known to Salmon as bastard spikenard (*Pharmacopoeia*). Hence lavender could be added 'to sweare by' by those who might cheat but would not risk swearing falsely.

3 Gallypots were small earthen glazed pots used by apothecaries for ointments and medicines (OED).

Whellan and I hope it will now come safe to you after all the mishaps that has attended it. I was forced to pay one half for Salvage as it was appraised which was 15s Please to deliver the Small Case to Mr Thomas Greaves upon demand hee paying his proportion of Freight: etc.

I have with this parcell sent you 4 Grosse of Gally potts which I find charged to your last Invoyce tho they were not then sent threw mistake and therefore I have not charged them now I have sent them[4]. There is noe good Spanish saffron[5] to bee gotten; I have waited in hopes of meeting with a parcell till I can stay noe longer for fear your Brother bee gone soe am forced to conclude my letter. But depend on it, if I can possibly meet with any before your Brother bee quite gone I deliver some to him under his owne perticuler care for the rest of the goods are shipt. If I should not, Capt Holland is put up for New England and I will not fayle of sending it by him; I hope it will bee somewhat cheaper if it prooves a good year for it. Allsoe then shall send some good Juniper berrys. Shall adde noe more but request you not fayle me in returns by the Mast Fleet remaine Sir   Yours   JC

43 MR THOMAS BARTON

London July 24 1712

SIR

This serves onely to inclose invoyce and bill of Loading of part of your order shipt in Capt Cary in the Severn Inn Gally. The remainder shall ship you in Capt Savage who suppose will sayle att the same time with the Mast Fleet; I was not willing to venture all in one bottom. Shall then write att large to you and remaine   Yours   JC

Sent per Capt Cary

44   [*Thomas Barton*]

Aug: 25: 1712

SIR

I am now arrived to the 25 August and this serves to inclose Invoyce and bill of Loading of the remainder of your Invoyce not sent before which I have

4 This sentence repeats one earlier in the letter exactly.
5 Spanish saffron was more highly regarded than English.

now sent by Capt Savage which I wish well to you and to your Content; everything is now sent accept the Lapis Bezoard which I have omitted by reason of the extravagant price of it it being above 5£ an ounce and scarce any to bee hade att that price neither. Allsoe the Butterbarr[1] and Masterwort[2] seeds each ½ ounce are not to bee gott; them plants are raised from slips and not from seed. I tryed to procure them but could not. Allsoe have sent but 4 ounces of Sweet Marjoram[3] seeds, it being very dear and they tell me 4 ounces is enough to plant a quarter of an Acre of ground; suppose you onely use it for your garden and if soe I am sure there is as much as you will need. There is noe Turbith in London, we use Jallops for it; nor noe good Juniper Berrys soe have sent but 3 lbs of them. I desyre you to deliver 2 lbs of the Spicknard you have by you to Mr Savage. He wrote to me for 2 lbs and there is none to be gott here; I could sell it now if I hade it here for 24s a pound; I wish you hade returned it before but wee expect some by every ship from East India, and then I suppose it will bee cheaper againe. I have carefully read over and pondered your long letter about your Currant money and tho after all I must owne I doe not well understand it yet me thinks there is such a tinge of honesty runs throw the whole that I cannot but owne I am throughly satisfyed with your proposalls and hope this will bee the last time there will ever bee occasion to have any disputes about it. And Therefore desyres if possible to make your returnes next year by Silver Coyn if possible to bee hade or by bills of Exchange if cannot bee in either of them, in Turpentine or oyle if cheape viz the Turpentine not exceeding 10s or 12s a hundred nor the oyle 20£ per Ton. I must leave it to you and desyre you to act for my interests as much as you can which I have noe reason to doubt of. I have advised Mr Savage of a large parcell of Druggs I designe to order to him from Jamaica. He

1 Butterbur, *Petasites vulgaris*, is a common English meadow plant, the root of which was used as a purgative and alexipharmic (Quincy *Complete English Dispensatory* 176; Grieve *Modern Herbal* 1: 148-9).

2 Masterwort, *Imperatoria ostruthium*, is a herb, the root of which was a purgative valued against poison, venomous bites, jaundice, and dropsies. It was a basic ingredient in plague water. Salmon warned (or was he really warning ?) 'It is not safe for Women with child, for it brings away the Birth with ease' (*Pharmacopoeia* 10, 59; Quincy *Complete English Dispensatory* 175-6). John Bartram commented that he had not seen this plant growing in any of the colonies. See his edition of Short *Medicina Britannica* 178.

3 Sweet marjoram, *Origanum marjorana*, is a common English aromatic herb used in cooking. A wide range of medicinal uses was given by Salmon including: dissolves congealed blood, swellings, and venomous bites; cures opium poisoning, toothache, coughs, and lung ailments. In Canary wine it helped relieve pains and griping of the bowels. Marjoram essence was valued for headaches, palsies, convulsions, and cramps. In Spanish wine the essence served as an antidote to poison, a stomach strengthener, and an aid in diseases of the spleen (Salmon *Pharmacopoeia* 66-7).

will I believe show you an Invoyce of them; if any of them bee what you want I have desyred him to deliver to you what quantity you please att the prices mentioned in the Invoyce. They were sent by order to a Gentleman there who was dead before they came thither and I cannot bring them back hither againe because the Parliament has a new duty upon all Druggs of 20 perCent which will considerably advance Druggs tho there should bee a peace, which wee are now in dayly expectation of. I have made the Elixir Salutis one 3rd part stronger than the last and have sent both these parcells in Trunkes as you advised me. What you call Grocery I have sent some but not soe much as you writ for because Sulphur is very dear now and Starch is risen a 1d a pound since the last 28 lbs I bought. I hope if there bee a peace things will be better settled before next spring. There was some roome left in the Trunk which I filled up with empty violls, which I suppose can bee noe burden to you. I desyre you to deliver the inclosed to Mr Thomas Greaves when you have opertunity. I was forced to crosse out the Saffron out of the Invoyce not being able to gett good it being extravagant dear to but wee hope quickly it will bee cheaper and then shall not fayle you by first ship. Remaine with etc.   JC

45 TO MR EMERSON[1] ATT NEW CASTLE IN NEW ENGLAND

July 25 1712

SIR

I have yours last spring per Mast Fleet wherein you complane of the Dearnesse of the Medicin you hade of me and allsoe advise me you hade sent 3£ 10s in part by Capt Martin; as to the first I shall onely say they were as cheape as you could have bought them here with ready money, and for the other I expected especially from a man of your Coat that you would not have put me off with such a foolish sham for when I come to talk with Capt Martin he possitively affirmed he hade noe such order from you nor hade he any money of yours in his hands, nor none have I received from him. I must let you know that I cannot but highly resent such treatment and thinke it is highly

---

1 John Emerson (1670-1732), son of Rev. John Emerson of Gloucester, Mass., graduated from Harvard in 1689. He preached at Manchester (1695-8), Salem, and Ipswich (1703) before accepting an invitation to become the first minister at Newcastle, near Piscataqua. He visited England in 1708, returning to Newcastle, where he preached until March of 1715 when he became pastor of South Church, Portsmouth, New Hampshire (Sibley *Harvard Graduates* 3: 418-21; Savage *Genealogical Dictionary* 2: 117; Sewall *Diary* 2: 284; 3: 356).

unbecomeing the Character you beare. I hade much rather you should have sayd nothing about it then shuffle soe for I can call it noe better, and I hope I shall learne att last to bee wiser then trust my effects abroad where I allways meet with disapoyntments. This comes by way of Mast Fleet and I desyre and expect you will make the full returnes by the returne of the same and [not?] give me the uneasy Task of writing againe. Expecting your complyance herewith, shall adde noe more but remaine etc.   JC

Sent another Coppy per Capt Savage Aug: 25, 1712

46 MR WILLIAM LITTLE

London Aug 25 1712

SIR

I received both yours per Fleet but am att a great losse how to judge of your management; you therein advertize[1] me you hade shipt a large quantity of goods on board Capt Kent and because you were unwilling to risque the whole earnestly pressed me to gett you a hundred pound ensured on her, and in case you did not come over in her yourself as you writ you design to doe, you would consigne the goods to me. Now upon your request you might reasonably expect I should act accordingly and therefore applyed myself to the insureing offices to gett it done but found them very unwilling to meddle they objecting she was a small foole and might bee pickt up by the least privateer; I offered att first 12 Guineys perCent which was the least any one I could understand hade done it for but could not gett it done. I then advanced gradually to 16 guineys but could not gett it done and in short being unwilling to venture higher it was not done att all. And as the sequell prooved it was well it was not done for when hee arrived I expecting either to see or heare from you pursuant to what you writt; I did neither and afterwards inquireing of Capt Kent about it was informed you shipt nothing upon him, allsoe that hee supposed you did not designe to come. Now how to reconcile these transactions with any prudent management is more than I am able to doe. Surely you should have been fully resolved to Ship your goods before you hade given me possitive orders to ensure which I hade certainely done if it hade been possible and then what a vast charge hade you brought upon yourself and a deale of trouble you hade given me for I spent some scores of Journeys about

---

1 Used here in the sense of calling another's attention to something (OED; Susie I. Tucker *Protean Shape: A Study in Eighteenth-Century Vocabulary and Usage* [London 1967] 189)

it and did more in it than I should have done hade the case been my owne and, when a report was spread about that the Ship was taken, I thinke my concerne and trouble for you was as great as if my owne interest hade been concerned. Besides your thus writeing has drawne on another Inconvenience for as I hinted in my last letter I designed to shipp your trunk a second time on Capt Whellan; But understanding you designed to come hither forbid the Shipping of it And ordered it back to London againe hopeing it might meet you here but it is not yet come; what the reason is I know not But have the farther Bad news to informe you of that while the Trunk lay in the Warehouse it was broke open and all the Brasse Drops[2] taken away and Severall of the Bookes which is a great misfortune but I know noe way to help it. I have demanded satisfaction of the person I paid the Salvage to but can gett noe redresse and I thinke it not worth Commenceing a law suit which would run out double the Charge and it may bee gett nothing by it neither. When the Trunk comes to me I shall keepe it till I either see you or heare from you for I know not how to act in this affayre being soe intricate. I desyre you to deliver the inclosed to your Brother the first opertunity. Remaine with hearty service Yours   JC

Sent by Capt Savage in Caswell Friggatt

Jan: 23: 1712/13

Wrote to Mr Savage by Capt Holland and advised him that by the next Ship I designed to send his Invoyce. Wrote allsoe att the same time and by the same conveyance to Mr Thomas Barton and advised him of the receipt of his letters and moneys etc.

47 MR CONRADE ADAMS

London Feb 27 1712/13

SIR

Yours of Aug 22 1712 came safe with the 6 Terazes[1] of Sugars per Capt Potts very safe and prooved very good and fitt for my owne proper use and I desyre if possible that some of your next remittances may bee in such att least 2 or 3

2 See above, letter 12.

1 A tierce is a cask containing one third of a standard measure (OED). In this case a tierce is a third of a Barbados hogshead of sugar, or approximately 335 lbs.

Terses. Allsoe received your Invoyces from Dr Jemmett and Mr Phyllips both which have complyed with and forwarded by this Conveyance and inclosed is Invoyce and bill of Loading of the same which I wish well to your hand and to their compleat satisfaction which I have endeavoured by takeing all possible care about the goodnesse and package of them. I was a little surprized att your mentioning in your letter that you had sent all the effects but you hade noe orders which seemes strange because I writ to you by severall Shipps last year and earnestly pressed you for a perticuler reason to send in Potts,[2] a coppy of which letters shall inclose that you may see what I then wrote. If they miscarryed I cannot help it but tis much they all should for I sent a Coppy of the same by Capt Winter, Capt Plumsted and Capt Potts. But if I hade sent none I thought what you writ the year before hade been sufficient, for you then possitively promised by the first fleet the next spring to make remittances. But I hope will by Capt Potts if you have done it before send the Ballance of my account; I hade rather have it by him than any other Ship if it can bee for hee is a very carefull honest man. And Now wee are like to have a peace (such a one as it is) suppose Ships will bee going to and fro often and not stay for Convoys and Fleet as they were forced formerly to doe and hope Freight will bee cheaper and Trade more incourageing and I hope if I live (by your interest) I may bee able to ingage farther in trade and make up my losses which you know have been great great [sic], tis now neare 20 yeares since I have traded with your Brother and yourself and I would very gladly still continue soe to doe. What I have farther to write about my Uncle Johnson is this; perceiveing you have not returned his effects last yeare, That his circumstances are worse than ever and therefore hee is forced to make over his debt to my sister and I would intreat you if possible to Ship his effects on Capt Potts and advise me of it that I may know it as soon as hee dos that my sister may attach it in his hands for she has lost all she has by his fayling. No 4 is a Trunk of Shooes which a Freind of mine[3] has sent as a tryall haveing a mind to venture a little abroad; hee will write to you himself and therefore need say noe more of that now. Shall write againe by other Ships remaine etc.

48 DR JEMMETT

London March: 2d 1712/13

SIR

Your order and Invoyce came safe to me under Covert of Mr Conrade Adams which I have taken perticuler care about and have sent them in Capt

2 The vessel captained by Captain Richard Potts; see above, letter 31.
3 A Mr Brookes; see below letter 60.

Richard Potts which I wish well to you and may prove to your full satisfaction. I have observed your direction in every thing onely whereas you order them to bee packt in a New Trunk I have packt the finest and lightest of the Dry things in a Trunk because I did not know but you might have need of it for your owne proper use but noe trunk would have held them all therefore have packt the remainder of them in a case. Allsoe you write for 2 ounces of oyl of Rhodium;[1] now the comon sort is what is most used because the finest is soe very Dear, therefore I have sent one ounce of each that you may for the future order which you please; the finest is cheaper conciderably then it use to bee. The last I bought of it cost me 28s an ounce. I consulted the best I could about the Booke and hope it will please you; I am informed tis the best that is extant of that kind. I hope all things will bee soe agreable to you as may incourage a yearly correspondance with you which I shall bee glad off and bee assured you shall have all the fayr and Candid dealing you can desyre or expect from   Yours

49 MR WILLIAM PHYLLIPS

London Mar 2, 1712 [/13]

SIR

I am favoured with yours of Aug 20 last with inclosed Invoyce for a Parcell of Druggs, Medicines etc. which I have forwarded to you by Capt Potts which hope will arrive safe to you and to your full Content and Satisfaction. I allsoe received the Tortoiseshell[1] by Capt Potts, and have gott you such a case made of it as you desyred; I tooke all the care I possibly could about and gave the necessary directions and I think it is a very neat one and every way exactly answearing your directions and I think all the Instruments are of the best sort. Allsoe the Medicines are all exactly according to your order accept only the Gascoyne Powder[2] which I have sent you without Bezoar that being now very much used by our Physicians and Bezoar being soe extravagantly dear that I cannot make it with the Bezoar but it will stand me in 16s an ounce or

---

1 Oil of rhodium, rosewood oil, was described by Salmon as the oil of Alpine rosewood, taken internally for palsies and kidney stones, but also a perfume and 'now of great use for that purpose' (*Pharmacopoeia* 414). Cruttenden's 'comon sort' was probably not made of Alpine rosewood.

1 The horny back plates of *Chelonia imbricata*, the smallest of the sea turtles, constitute this prized commodity. Carefully worked with heat and pressure, they are formed into boxes, combs, etc.
2 See above, letter 14, note 1. Surely Gascoigne's powder without bezoars would not be esteemed Gascoigne's powder at all.

very neare, and I was afraid you would thinke that to deare. I dare say you will find very little difference in the use of it where there is one ounce of that with Bezoar used here there is 3 of this sort which has every thing in it but the Bezoar. I thought it necessary to give you these hints. Allsoe the case being to large I have putt up more of the Empty Violls then you ordered which suppose can bee noe disadvantage to you. I shall bee allways ambitious of your Correspondance and value your Aquaintance and whatever you or your sons shall want shall allways carefully bee sent by Sir   Yours

50 TO MR THOMAS PERKINS ATT JAMAICA

Aprill 8 1713

SIR

I have received noe letter from you this 17 or 18 Months; still expecting by every Ship to heare from you and have still deferred writeing to you in hopes I should att last heare from you. Indeed considering how many fleet and running Shipps have come since your last I cannott but thinke it a strange neglect in you never to write. You cant but thinke it must bee a very great uneasynesse to me to thinke of such a large Cargoe to lye there 2 yeares togather and can heare nothing what is become of them. I know not what to thinke of it can hardly perswade myself you would take noe care about them after you hade promised you would, and yet on the other hand thinke it very strange you should give noe account whether they are sold or not or any part of them; Tis a very hard case to Trust ones effects abroad and have them soe neglected, for I cannot call it otherwise. My desyre therefore and positive order is if you have not disposed of them there nor if there bee not a certainety of your disposeing of them that you would by the first opertunity Shipp them for New England and Consigne them to Mr Habijah Savage Apothecary att Boston in New England. If you have sold none of them send as they were in the Same Package, if any are disposed of Send the remainder and take a perticuler account of what they are and send the Invoyce with them that I sent to you and write to Mr Savage that you did it by my direction and I have allsoe writ to him to let him know that I have ordered such things for him, and pray fayle not by the first opertunity to advise me what you have done, and let me have the perticulers of the former account which you never yet sent me and what you left in Mr Fernly hands which I never yet received. Sure you thinke abroad wee can live on the ayr here, to let things run on 4 or 5 yeares without Ballanceing accounts; pray let there bee an end put to it that I may know what I have to trust to and may have noe more uneasynesse about it. I can never Believe but you might have disposed of the goods the most of them att least being such Substantiall goods as must bee wanted if you hade been diligent in the matter, but you don't doe as you would be done by. I desyre you to concider of this matter allsoe; pray inquire of Mr Fernly what hee has done about Spaines debt for I never could gett any of it heare as he pretended I should. Remaine Yours   JC

51 MR THOMAS BARTON

London Apr: 9: 1713

SIR

Yours of Dec. 29 1712 per Ship Chester I am favoured with, with Bill of Exchange on Mr Loyd for 27£ 2s as allso a Bill on Capt Davis for 11£ both which Bills I have received as allsoe the Gold and Silver per Man of Warr for all which returne you my hearty thankes. This serves to inclose Invoyce and Bill of Loading of your order sent by this conveyance in the Amity Capt Thomas which wish well and safe by our hand and to your universall satisfaction which I have endeavoured. Have sent all now which was omitted before. I have allsoe concidered the contents of your letter and complyed with what you mention, being willing if possible that you may lye under noe discouragements tho I see noe prospect of goods beeing like to bee cheaper then they are here by the peace; what they may bee abroad I know not but for all sorts of Druggery it is dearer by 15 perCent att least then it was before the late tax upon it and peace is not like to mend it for the duty upon it being soe very large will more then Ballance the lessening of the Freight. I approve well of your prudent management of returnes which I beleive the best you could have done and if silver be not to bee hade for the future, I think Bills of Exchange are better then any goods at present; if any alterations happen to allter my thoughts, shall allwayes advice you of it as opertunity serves. As to what you mention of my makeing a mistake in the account to my owne disadvantage for which you claime a hat, I have herewith sent you one whether it prove as you mention or not, which hope you will accept. But as to what you charge me with in not giveing you credit for the Sperma Cocti I assure you it is a mistake for I have done as you will see by the Ballance of your account now sent Debtor and Creditor which hope will prove to your satisfaction. I shall endeavour allways to consult your Interest and advantage in every thing and comply with your perticuler orders, and hope to continue and increase our correspondance.[1] Have inclosed your account which I hope agrees with yours; This is as it att present stands in my Booke. As to what you write about Sperma Coeti the same as before, I believe if you send it, it will turne to a pretty good account; tis now worth refined 36s a pound and wee give such a weight to the refiners and they deliver back half as much but I am inclined to thinke if it bee as good as the last was it will yeild 20s a pound. How farr the duty may clog it I cannot say for tis 4s in the pound for all Druggs as they are rated in the Booke of rates but how much a pound that is valued att I cannott certainely tell. Desyre if money bee not to bee had to make returnes in Bills of Exchange or Turpentine if cheape, leave it to your prudent management am with etc.   Yours   JC

52 MR HABIJAH SAVAGE

Apr: 16 1713

SIR

Yours of Aug. 1 and Dec. 29 last are both before me and I diligently observe their contents: I have received allsoe your Bills on Mr Chalk for 100£ Sterling and on Mr Prince for 50£ Sterling and the 83 ounces Plate by Man of warr and 80£ of Mr Blettsoe but the other 20£ soe farr as I can understand is never like to bee paid. Mr Blettsoes man tells me his Master Despayred of getting it; others persons are in the same case. Noe doubt hee has given you an account of the matter soe twill bee needlesse to write any more about that. For all these payments and your great care therein I thinke myself greatly obliged to you and returne you my hearty thanks. I alsoe received your Invoyce which I have putt up and forwarded to you by this Conveyance the Amity Capt Thomas which I heartily wish well to you and may prove to your universall satisfaction. I have sent every thing in your order and what few things were left behind before. I have carefully and not without concernes observed all the discouragements you observe you have laine under and to give you an infallible proof how ready I am to doe anything that may make you easye and to prevent any complaints for the future, I have complied with your desyre and have charged you but 65 perCent advance for the whole accept 5 or 6 things which you never disputed and have altered my Booke and taken off what you objected against and have your account in my Booke to this day Debtor and Creditor as by the inclosed account here sent will appeare; soe

---

1 JC intended to finish here, but later crossed out 'remaine Yours JC.'

that I cannott see for the future how wee can ever have any difference or dispute but I have done all this to make you easye. I must take liberty to say I
cannott see any reason why Druggs bought well and with ready money
should not allow the same advance as if a man layd out his money in Woolen
or Linen Cloth which you know sells for more advance a great deale, but I
shall write not about that. What advantages wee may reap by peace (which
att last wee have gott), in generall I know not but I can see noe manner of
reason to thinke any sort of Druggs will bee cheaper concidering the vast duty
layd on them by which allmost every thing is advanced 20 perCent. Indeed
Freight must bee cheaper but the duty will much more then Ballance that.
The tryall must prove what alterations it will produce. You complaine of my
neglect in not giveing possitive orders about returns, now I doe not see how I
can well doe that nor what need there is of it if I could, when I have soe prudent a person to deale with. You upon the spott know what things may bee
bought well better then I can, besides things vary soe strangely; a year agoe
Turpentine bore a great price and they that hade it made more then Sterling
of it, now tis fallen above half; soe that I cannot see how I can give possitive
directions but must referr myself to your prudent Conduct onely. If money or
Bills of exchange can bee hade any thing reasonable hade rather have that,
there being lesse trouble in them but if not you may send what Comoditys
your Countrys affords. I doe not know but what you mention of Bottoming
some ship[1] may doe very well but if you doe I desyre if possible you would advice of it before hand that I may make insurance which now on the peace I
suppose will bee much lower; as to any part of a New Ship I desyre you not to
doe anything in that for I have been concerned in a great many and have lost
by all and would scarce accept of a part in any ship if it were offered me gra-
tis and bee obliged to keepe it; and therefore I can referr myself to you and
desyre you would not expect any other or more perticuler orders. I shall endeavour for the future never to omitt anything in your orders.

53 MR THOMAS GREAVES OF CHARLES TOWNE NEW ENGLAND

Apr: 16 1713

SIR

Yours of December 26 last past I have received and your Invoyce which I

---

1 OED records no verbal form of 'bottom' comparable to the verb 'to bottomry' meaning to lend a
shipowner money on the security of the ship, with lenders bearing risks.

have complyed with and sent you in the Amity Capt Thomas, And inclosed is Invoyce and bill of Loading of it which I wish well to your hands and to you content. I have put up the best of every thing and charged them as low as possible being willing to give you all incouragement to procure and establish a further Correspondance yearly, and shall allways bee ready to serve you the uttmost of my power. Remaine   Yours   JC

Note: wrote att the same time to Mr Emerson att Ipswich and advised him I hade received the whole of his Bill.

Wrote allsoe att the same time to Mr Jackson pressing him to make speedy returnes.

54 MR WILLIAM LITTLE

London July 25 1713

SIR

The last I am favoured with from you is of the 9th of January last giveing me the Melancholly news of your Brothers[1] death for which I am heartyly concerned as allsoe that you designed to Shipp on his account 20 Barrells of Turpentine and 8 on your owne account on Capt Leverett: which 28 Barrells are safe arrived but received not one letter with them hade neither Bill of Loading nor Invoyce neither by him nor any other Ship since, tho wee have hade 2 or 3 Shipps arrived since him; it was a strange neglect in you. It was a wonder I ever hade the Turpentine for I hade noe claime to it but by virtue of the letter above mentioned which would not have been sufficient to demand hade not the Ship been consigned to a Freind of mine. Alsoe must advice you of a farther and greater omission in not sending a certificate along with it, for want of that I can make noe claime to the Queens Bounty which is allowed to incourage the importing of it. I have taken all the precaution possible to secure it provided you send a certificate with all speed. Your Merchants will direct you how to doe it; you must make Oath before some one of your Magistrates that such a day of the Month and year you shipt 28 Barrells of Turpentine on such a Ship and Master consigned to me being the Growth of New England etc. Your Merchants will direct you it and this certificate you

---

1 Thomas Little died at Plymouth, Mass., 22 December 1712 (Sibley *Harvard Graduates* 4: 253).

must send over by the first oppertunity which I must show to the Commissioners of the Navy and that will intitle me to the Bounty which otherwise cannot bee obtained.[2] Therefore pray doe not neglect it. I have put it up in a Warehouse and not sold it for att the present it is not above 12s a hundred. I hope it will advance tho manny people are of opinion it will not; I know it has been sold for 11s a hundred since this came in. As soon as any incouragement apeares will dispose of it and give your Brothers account and yours Credit for the produce of it and as soon as possible transmit it to you. I perceive by yours of the above date you received mine of the 25th of August wherein I fully informed you of the manny misfortunes of your Trunk. What I have farther now to adde is that the Trunk is sent back from Plymouth hither and upon my opening found as I hinted before all the Brasse Wares gone and Severall of the Bookes stole and of those that remained severall of them and these the Best damaged extreamly by the Salt Water, which damag when it hapned to them I cannot learne. I have done all that is possible to gett some allowance and am promised I shall have it but how much I cannott tell but I feare not near enough to make good the damage. Depend on it I will doe what ever I can in it and as soon as ever I can doe it will send the Trunk againe, I hope to doe it within a Month. I am heartyly sorry for such a series of disapoyntments but I can noe way help it and as I hinted to you before it is chiefly owing to your self[3] that you hade not the trunk shipt on Capt Whellam, which would have saved me a great deale of trouble and vexation which I have hade about it more then ever I hade in any such trifling affayr in my whole life: This is the needful etc.

55

Oct: 3: 1713

Wrote him againe by the Providence Capt Dawson and sent Coppy of the forementioned and pressed him not to neglect forwarding will all speed the Certificate for the Turpentine. Allsoe advised him that by the same Ship hade sent his Trunck of Bookes and inclosed Bill of Ladeing for them: advised there was wanting 3 Bookes and the Brasse wares viz 3rd volume of Col-

---

2 On the bounty scheme of 1705 and its evolution see Joseph J. Malone *Pine Trees and Politics* (Seattle 1964) 10-27.

3 JC changed 'your owne neglect' to 'yourself' here.

lyers Essays[1] 2nd volume Brittish Empyre in America[2] and 1 volume of Rapins workes[3] which promised to put up the next time I sent any goods to Mr Savage.

56 TO MR HABIJAH SAVAGE BY THE PROVIDENCE CAPT DAWSON

Oct: 3: 1713

SIR

I am favoured with your of May 5 1713, wherein you advice of a Bill of 100£ Sterling you have forwarded via Newfoundland which I have yet heard nothing of but hope I Shall ere long. I thanke you for your care in that and all former remittances; I hope the Goods last sent in Capt Thomas came safe and to your content. And you may depend if God spare life and health shall never fayle for the future in complying with your Invoyce in every perticuler since you mention it is soe detrimental to you, but I really did it as I thought for the best, for when a thing is extravagantly scarce and dear wee generally send lesse then is writt for, but shall not doe soe againe by your order. Tho have not materiall busynesse was not willing to slip this oppertunity of paying my gratefull respects to you. I am Yours   JC

57 TO MR THOMAS PERKINS ATT JAMAICA

Dec: 12 1713

SIR

After waiting 2 years for a letter I was att last favoured with yours of Aug 6 last by the Heroine Gally advising you hade sold my goods for 200£ to Dr

1 Best known for his *A Short View of the Immorality and Profaneness of the English Stage* (London 1698), Jeremy Collier (1650-1726), nonjuror and church historian, published *Essays upon Several Moral Subjects*, the first two parts of which went through six editions by the time the four-part work was fully published in 1709 (DNB; Rose Anthony *The Jeremy Collier Stage Controversy, 1698-1726* [New York 1937] *passim*; Joseph Wood Krutch *Comedy and Conscience after the Restoration* 2nd ed [New York 1949] esp. 101-49, 264-72).

2 John Oldmixon *The British Empire in America* 2 vols. (London 1708)

3 René Rapin, SJ (1621-87), neo-classical literary critic and historian of the Jansenist movement. Numerous Dutch editions of his works appeared in the forty years after his death. William Little may well have ordered the two-volume English translation 'by several hands,' *The Whole Critical Works of Monsieur Rapin* (London 1706). That is the edition that is included in *Harvard College Library Catalogue of 1723* (Boston 1723) 92. See E.T. Dubois's introduction to Rapin's *Les Réflexions sur la Poétique de ce Temps* (Geneva 1970) vii-xxxv.

Tredway with a promise I should have account of Sales by Capt Topsam and the returnes by the next ship after him; which was very pleaseing news to me till Capt Topsam arrived and noe letter by him and 4 or 5 Shipps more since are come in and not one Line. This I confesse astonished me and the best sense it can possible beare is that you are a wonderfull negligent man; you must Imagine it must raise strange jealousys in anyone to bee soe dealt by. I would have you remember that tho you are att a great distance from me and soe may thinke yourself secure yet the eye of God is upon you and you must give an account to him. I am unwilling to entertaine hard thought of you but I cannot well help beleiveing you are not the man I tooke you for; And in short I must let you know that if I have not some satisfactorry account from you before Capt Madden sayles I must thinke of some way to right myself for I assure you cannot beare such losses. I have my whole life suffered by being kind to others and tis time now to have regard to myself and my numerous famyly, I shall be well pleased if an accouunt comes before I send againe that may disapoynt my thoughts in that respect. If any accident hade hapned that you could not by any one Ship send the account there have been soe many have come away since that tis impossible but you might if you would have sent it by some or other of them. I still hope to hear some better news from you which may give me reason still to beleive you are an honest man. Your Freind   JC

[*in margin*: Sent by the Soloman]

58 TO MR SAMUEL PROCTER ATT ANTEGO

Jan: 8 1713/14

SIR

The last letter I am favoured with of yours is of July 23 1711, now near 18 Months agoe wherein you excuse your not haveing yet sent the ballance of my account and desyre I would have a Charitable opinion of you till I saw cause to the contrary. I would bee very cautious of censureing any person but att the same time cannott but judge 7 yearcs a great while for a person to bee out of his money the Comon Interest would come to allmost half the sume in that time. I have diligently lookt over all your letters (2 of which I have by this conveyance sent back to you that you may bee satisfyed the bearer came from me and is noe Impostor) and by the account therein mentioned have drawne out an Account Current herein inclosed by which you are Debtor to me in Antegua money 111£ 12s 4¼d which Ballance I intreat you would not fayle of Shipping by the Bearer hereof Capt Samuell Galpine who is my perticuler Freind and whose receipt shall bee a full discharge for whatever hee receives from you. Hee is a person I suppose well knowne to you and therefore begg you will not fayle this oppertunity for indeed I greatly want the money and I cannot but thinke you must owne it is more then time it was paid. Your complyance herein will greatly oblige   Yours etc.   JC

59 DR ROBERT ANDERSON ATT BARBADOS

Jan 23 1713/14

SIR

I am favoured with yours bearing date Oct 6 last past and am glad to hear of your safe arrivell there and of your prospect of incouragement as allsoe for any good effects my letter of recommendation to Mr Adams has hade and wish it may still have a greater. Allsoe observe your Invoyce of Medicines you want and have by this conveyance Capt Lassells Shipt them as apeares by the inclosed Invoyce and bill of loading which I heartyly wish well to your hand and hope they will every way prove to your full satisfaction. I have charged you the very lowest price and (which is the Method of dealing to the Leeward Islands) 50 per cent advance if payd in goods and I stand to the losse of them which is generally near 40 per cent losse; I send a parcell by this very Ship to Mr Adams which hee agreed for upon the same termes, I mention this because perhaps you may bee a stranger to the Method of dealing to those parts. I would not in the least impose on you or take any advantage of you if it were in my power but hope to incourage a farther Correspondance and shall allways bee ready to supply you with what you want and upon the most reasonable termes and if you meet with any person there that deales in my way would bee glad of your recommendation. I have putt up a packett of letters in the Chest and have inclosed one in this; the Chest was not bigg enough to hold all the Violls but hope these may serve you for the present till the next opertunity of sending to you. I shall take perticuler care to forward any orders I may att any time receive from you. This is the needfull att present but etc from Sir   Yours   JC

Sent by Capt Robert Lassells

60 TO MR CONRADE ADAMS AND COMPANY ATT BARBADOS

Jan: 23 1713/14

SIR

I have been favoured with manny letters from you within a few Months past as allsoe Invoyce and Bill of loading for 16 hoggsheads of Sugar per Capt Potts which arrived safe and proved good and came to a pretty good markett for which and all former favours I returne you hearty thanks. Allsoe received the Invoyce from you for Dr William Phyllips which I have by this conveyance Capt Lassells forwarded to you as per inclosed invoyce and Bill of Loading fully apeares, which I wish well to you and hope they will prove to his intyre satisfaction. Inclosed is a letter from my Freind Mr Brookes who sent you the small Trunk of Shooes; hee is att present through some indisposition gone into the Country soe when you make his returnes you may please to consigne it to me which hee desyred me to act for him haveing noe famyly here. Alsoe inclosed is a letter from my uncle Major Johnson. Both parcells of Sugars you sent in Sherburne and Waldye came into my hands and I made shift to secure one half of the produce of them for my poor ruined sister And begg when you send the remainder it may bee done in the same manner that I may have timely notice of it. The Terse of first whites were very good indeed, I bought them my self for my owne use; I wish if you could once a year when you make my returnes I might have such a tearse as the best of them was for my owne use. I allsoe received your account of Sales and account Current which I have noe reason to question but cannott reconcile it with mine. You make yourself Debtor to me but 6-0-10¾ but my account makes you 29-5-5¾. You may remember I gave you an account Feb 28 last whereby you were Debtor 283:18:3½ And the goods you sent this year per Capt Potts amounted to but 254-12-9¾ soe that by that account there must remaine 29-5-5¾. I thought I was very carefull in the Account and you makeing noe objections against it I thought you hade been satisfyed about it. If it dos not apear playne to you I shall bee willing to bee convinced if I am in an errour and I am well satisfyed you will not insist upon any thing but what is just and fayr. I intreat the favour to deliver the inclosed to Mr Phyllips with the goods. Allsoe I take notice with great concerne what you write about Dr Jemmett; I hope when hee conciders the matter hee will send againe and I intreat you to use your endeavours to soften him, and I promise to doe all lyes in my power to encourage him, therefore shall hope to heare from him againe and shall bee glad of any other Invoyces you can procure for me. Perticulerly I thanke you for your kindnesse to my Freind Mr Anderson which hee has owned to me has been great, I hope hee will endeavour to merritt your favours. This is the needful etc.

Sent by Capt Lascelles

London Feb: 18: 1713/4

SIR

Yours of Dec. 8 last per her Majestys Ship Reserve I am favoured with the inclosed bills of Loading in all Amounting to 114£ 3s 0d as allsoe advice of your shipping 5 Ton of Loggwood in the Rebecca Friggott which is not yet arrived hope in time she will; for all these favours (with all former ones)[1] I send you my hearty thanks. Alsoe inclosed is an Invoyce of your small parcell you lately writt for, the Box being soe very small, I was afraid it should bee lost if sent alone and therefore have putt it up in Mr Bartons case there being just roome for it. I thought it best, soe to do. I have desyred him to deliver it to you; you may easyly compute the Charges which cant bee much; it comes by this conveyance Capt Thomas. I hope shortly to receive a larger Invoyce from you which shall bee carefully forwarded to you by first opertunity. The Loggwood if it arrives safe will come but to an indifferent Markett however I heartyly thanke you and beeleive still tis as good as any returnes in goods is but it is 5 or 6 pound a Ton cheaper then it was 6 month agoe; some are of the opinion it will rather mend then grow worse. Mr Barton advises me he delivered you 2 lbs of Spicknard, att 24s per lb New England money, which I have charged to your account; now that is worth 3 pound Sterling a pound here, now it is worth indeed any price there not being 10 lbs of [it] in England. I often wish't for the 6 lbs Mr Barton hade of me here if that would doe: it cost me 18s a pound tho I charged him but 12s because it was a little dull att that time. Soe your account as it stands now is 384-10-11½ of which you have remitted 273-0- soe remaines due to Ballance 111-10-11½ in New England money. I hope I shall receive the Bills when they become due without much trouble tho the persons they are drawne upon live att such a wide distance will make it somewhat troublesome. If any of them should not bee paid shall advise you of it per Capt Sherburne who will sayle in lesse then a Month by which time shall I hope bee able to give you some account of the Loggwood. Therefore shall adde noe more but remaine with Tenders of my Service etc.

JC

---

1 Closing parenthesis added

62 MR THOMAS BARTON

London Feb: 18 1713/4

SIR

Yours of Nov. 19 and Dec. 9 last I am favoured with as allsoe the 176 ounces Silver by her Majestys Ship reserve being in full Ballance of all your Accounts which I acknowledge myself fully paid and satisfyed and hereby Returne you my hearty thanks for this and all former favours. The 1-15-8½ overplus I have according to your order sent in Holmans Ink powder:[1] viz 3 Quarters of a Grosse; it is 48s a Grosse. Allsoe by this conveyance have sent your Invoyce. You will find in the case a small Box or Case directed for Mr Savage which intreat the favour to deliver to him who will pay you Proportionably for the Freight. Inclosed is Invoyce and Bill of Loading for the Parcell now sent in the Amity, Capt Thomas. I wish them well and safe to your content. Indeed after all our great expectations from peace I don't see but Druggs are like to bee Dearer; the new duty of 4s in the pound ruines all and the Duty is layd on them according to the value that was putt upon them in the booke of Rates 50 yeares agoe wherein manny things were soe valued that the duty is more upon them then they are now worth. Wee have some small hopes and there will bee some attempt to gett it eased this Parliament but question whether they will make any thing of it. Gambooge is now worth neare 20s a pound for to buy in parcell and manny other things are extravagantly deare; indeed all that helps out is Freight is cheaper or else Drugs in generall would bee above 10 percent dearer then before the peace. I have lookt over all your accounts and find I gave you Creditt for the Sperma Coeti Apr 18 1710 7£ 16s which must bee New England money not sterling for it was charged att 28s a pound and 12s was deducted for Freight and charges brought it to 7£ 16. I entered the Catalogue being in a paper by itself and did not observe your observe about viol Corkes, till I came to looke over your letters againe in order to answear them when I found it. I am sorry for it for hade I seen it I could have putt in some into the vacancys but the Chest fitting soe exact it would not have held many and there was roome for noe paper att all; hope the Disapoyntment will not bee great. The oyl of Spike now sent is as good, I am confident, as any in London, and sent in Bottles. This is the needfull at present but etc. JC

---

1 In an inventory of the estate of Boston bookseller Michael Perry made in 1700, 2 lb of Holman's ink powder was valued at 1s (*Publications of the Prince Society* 4 [Boston 1867]: 318).

63 MR JAMES HENDERSON CHYRURGEN OF THE SEAFORD MAN OF WARR ATT NEW YORK

Mar: 13 1713/14

SIR

Inclosed is a letter to you from Mr Richard Borman who was my apprentice 8 yeares[1] and he, haveing left his busynesse of[f], shewed me your letter and askt me if I were willing to send you the goods you ordered from him and upon the fayr account hee gave of you and being incouraged allsoe by your Freind Mrs Jackson, I have Shipt them in the Drake Capt Tucker. Inclosed is Invoyce and Bill of Loading of the same which I wish well to your hands and to your content. I have observed your directions in packing with Tow[2] and hope they will come very safe. The Compounds are all put up in the same Quantitys (or as near as the vessells would hold) as you ordered but some of the Druggs being very scarce and deare have put up somewhat a less Quantity of but hope they will answear your purpose for the present. You may have larger Quantitys any time upon your advice and I assure you, you shall find very Candid usage att all times from me and indeed it was in hopes of a farther correspondance that I made this beginning my busynesse lyes much wholesale beyond sea and am sure I can afford you as cheap and good as any one can. All the objection Mrs Jackson made was what if the things should bee lost before they arrived to you, in answeare to that I assured her I would ensure them to you; I hope you will not bee gone thence before they arrive and wish as these prove I may have farther dealings with you. Please by the first oppertunity after you receive them to give me advice thereof as allsoe when you shall remoove your station and whether and when you expect to come for England. This with hearty Service is the needfull from Sir   yours JC

[*in margin*: Direct for me att the Green Dragon in Newgate Street, London]

64 CAPT JOHN TUCKER COMANDER OF THE DRAKE ATT NEW YORK

Mar: 13 1713/14

SIR

By your leave and advice I write this that in case the Seaford Man of warr should bee gone from New York before your arrivall there or in case Mr Hen-

---

1 Richard Boreman, son of Richard Boreman of Westfield, Sussex, carpenter, was apprenticed to JC for eight years on 3 September 1700 (GL, MS 8200/4, 124).
2 Tow is coarse and broken bits of hemp (OED).

dersen the Surgeon of her should bee dead to whom a small case of Medicines
Shipt upon you is consigned; Then I intreat the favour of you to open my letter to him sent in your Bagge in which you will find the Invoyce which, if you
can dispose off to any Apothecary at New York, please to doe it; if not pray
Ship them by the first oppertunity for New England and consigne them to
Mr. Habijah Savage att Boston Apothecary who deals with me and send the
Invoyce with them and I shall advise him of it allsoe. But if you can sell them
att New York I must desyre you to remember the price charged in the Invoyce is but Sterling price and therefore if you sell them there must doe it
with proportionable advance for the discount of their money and please to lay
it out to the best advantage you can and bring it back with you which I shall
willingly give you commissions for and satisfye you every way. I hope there
will bee noe occasion for any of this trouble but I onely doe it out of caution
for feare Mr Henderson should bee gone or Dead or the like. Your favour
herein will greatly oblige   Your humble Servant   JC

65 MR THOMAS BARTON

London Apr: 22 1714:

SIR

I am favoured with yours of Jan. 18 1713 per Capt Brumsall with Invoyce
[*and*] a farther order for a small parcell of wares which I have forwarded to
you by this Conveyance, Capt Corney in the Sagamore Galley, which I wish
well and safe to your hands and that they may prove to your intyre content
and satisfaction. Inclosed is Bill of Loading and Invoyce of the same as allsoe
a 2nd Bill of Loading for those things sent you in Capt Thomas. I observe
what you desyre as to the prizes of Furrs, Castor Hepatick,[1] Aloes. For Furrs
they may doe pretty well if well bought. Aloes I beleive will doe as well as
anything onely the extreame high new duty ruines all; But if you can send it
over not exceeding 6£ perCent here without that duty I beleive it will turne
to a good account provided it don't fall again but Castorium is exceeding low
and pays a vast duty is not worth heare above 5s per lb. I see noe prospect of
lowering the Duty on Druggs and if it bee not busynesse will bee intyrely
ruined, manny Druggs that duty on them being more than they are worth
which is a very great hardship upon us. Druggs in generall have rise since the
peace att least 15 perCent and some things more then double as Rhubarb

---

1 Literally of the liver of beaver, *Castor hepatic* is another term for castoreum.

Cortex,[2] Rad Contrayerva,[3] etc soe that att present wee are in a farr worse condition then wee were before the peace. I have packt up your things with viol Corkes which were omitted before and have sent them in a Trunk. This is the needfull att present from Sir   Yours etc.

Sent by the Sagamore Galley.

66 MR THOMAS GREAVES

London Apr: 22 1714

SIR

Yours of Dec. 29 last past I am favoured with whereby you excuse your delay of payment soe long; I did indeed hope for and expect it this yeare. I thought small Bills of Exchange hade been easyer come by then larger. As to my ordering some person there to receive it I cannot thinke it soe proper but, to please you and hope to oblige you I have writt to my Freind Mr Habijah Savage Apothecary att Boston to receive it of you if you tender it to him and give you a full discharge. The sume is 26£-18s-7d. I am troubled you should prejudice your busynesse by not sending for what you want; therefore deferr not sending for what you have occasion which shall with all speed bee conveyed to you by Sir   Yours etc.

Sent by the Sagamore Galley

67 MR GEORGE JACKSON

London Aprill: 22 1714

SIR

Yours of Dec. 15 ultimate is before [me] the contents thereof take notice of; you there advice that you last year sent 20£ to North Brittaine by Capt Buck-

---

2 *Rhubarb cortex*, or rhubarb bark, is from an oriental herb, no relation to the vegetable of the same name. The drug was valued as an astringent or, in heavier doses, as a violent purgative used in jaundice and cases of worms in children (Quincy *Complete English Dispensatory* 192-4). It was also used in treatment of gonorrhea (Salmon *Pharmacopoeia* 15). Rhubarb was already expensive, especially since the Russian government established a monopoly on its westward transit after 1704 (*Ency. Brit.* 23: 273).

3 *Dorstenia contrayerva*, a plant native to tropical America, has a reddish brown root of bitter and pungent taste, valued as a stimulant, tonic, and antidote to snake bites, and as a perspiration inducer considered valuable in fevers (Quincy *Complete English Dispensatory* 171, 175; OED; Grieve *Modern Herbal* 1: 219).

lin of Boston in the George with orders to him to remittt the produce to me, as to that affayre I doe assure you I never heard a word of it before nor have I ever received one farthing from him or any one else on your account. It was very strange that att the same time you sent you did not give me advice of it that I might have sent to Glascow to enquire after it which I could easyly have done but now tis soe long since can't expect to heare anything of it; therefore must not looke upon any part of the Debt as satisfyed, But desyre you will not fayle this yeare to remitt the whole for you know tis 3 or 4 yeares since you hade the things and tis more then time it was discharged therefore pray fayle not and you'l oblige Sir   Yours etc.

Sent by the Sagamore Galley

68 MR HABIJAH SAVAGE

London Aprill 22 1714

SIR

Yours of Dec. 8 and Jan 18 last I am both favoured with with your Invoyce which I have forwarded to you by this conveyance Capt Corney in the Saga-more Galley which I wish well to your hands and to your full satisfaction which I have endeavoured all I can; have made very little alteration in any-things vizt instead of 20 lbs Rad Curcuma[1] have sent but 10 lbs by reason of the extravagant price of it it being now worth 5s a pound, and wee are in ex-pectation of some coming home next Ships from India then hope it will bee cheaper. In looking over your former account find I have charged you but 10d a pound for it, but that is noe new thing with us for manny sort of Druggs are risen proportionably. Cortex Peru[2] what I could have bought some time

1 The root of the South Asian herbacious perennial *Curcuma longa* or turmeric was used in the treat-ment of jaundice and dropsy, in addition to being a major ingredient in curry powder (Quincy *Complete English Dispensatory* 149; Salmon *Pharmacopoeia* 6, 45; OED; Grieve *Modern Herbal* 2: 882-3).

2 *Cortex peru*, cinchona bark or Jesuits' bark, is the bark of a tropical American evergreen. The bark, from which quinine would be isolated in the nineteenth century, was valued in the treat-ment of a wide variety of fevers and fluxes (Quincy *Complete English Dispensatory* 175). It was 1676 before the first English physician wrote supporting its use, and it was not, according to one au-thority, used in the English American colonies until late in the century (W.B. Blanton *Medicine in Virginia in the Seventeenth Century* [Richmond, Va. 1930] 113). Its use was not hastened by the prac-tice of selling black cherry bark made bitter by tincture of aloes as cortex Peru (Brooks *Sir Hans Sloane* 87). Josselyn's description of sassafras, including 'And why may not this be the bark the Jesuits powder was made of, that was so famous, not long since, in England, for agues?' (*New England's Rarities* 65), was no help either.

since for 25£ is now worth a 100£ and Rad Contrayerva which use to bee sold for 4s is now worth 20s and in Short Druggs in the whole are 15 or 20 perCent dearer then before the peace; the extravagant new duty ruines all. There is noe good Spanish Saffron in Towne; what is [*is*] 45s a pound And one pound of English is worth 3 lbs of it and therefore English being pretty reasonable I have sent 3 lbs of very fine English and noe Spanish att all which hope you will like better. There is one thing you write for vizt Fecula Aronis[3] which is not to bee hade in England I q[*uestion*] whether there bee an oz of it in the whole K[*ingdom*] but next month being the season to make it I will endeavour to send you some by the next conveyance tho I B[*elieve*] shall not bee able to gett a pound of it. What I have sent are very good and Cheape bought and considering you take large Quantitys have made noe difference but charged those bought with ready money att the same price with the Medicines vizt 65 perCent advance[4] which concidering the vast losse on returnes I thinke is to cheape in reason, concidering how great the losse is upon returnes but I am willing to give you all possible incouragement. I have received all your Bills except that for 7£ 5s which I cannot gett yet but I am in some hopes I shall. The Loggwood is att last come safe but to a miserable account; I have sold it but for 18£ 15s a Ton, and the dutys here with the wast upon stood me in very near 10£ a Ton and then I leave you to judge what a poor account it must turne to tho I lay noe blame on you but doubt not but you did it for the best and I returne you thankes for it. I thinke Bills of Exchange are better then any goods; [*blot*: I?] must leave it to your management and shall bee satisfyed with if prove well or ill; goods vary soe much, what bares a good price be fure can send and have any returnes it may bee fallen to one halfe. I have one favour to request of you vitz there is one Mr Thomas Greaves of Charles-Town owes me a small sume of 26£-18s-7d New England money which hee writes me word he cannott gett a Bill of Exchange small enough for but will pay it to any person I shall apoynt to receive it there. I have writ to him by this conveyance to pay it to you which I intreat you to receive and give him a full discharge from me and please to returne it to me with the next returnes you make either by Bill of Exchange or goods as you doe your owne. If I can save you as much in any affayr here I shall bee ambitious of it. Sir I hope if you send any more Loggwood it will bee at a Lower price for those that Deale it here tell me it use to bee bought in New England for 7£ a ton. I have carefully examined all the Account from the beginning and all I can find is as I sent it before April 16 171[*blot*: 3?]. By an account rendered from you which I

---

3 Salmon describes a faecula of Aron root (golden rod), the sediment from the juice of bruised and pressed roots, as opening the bowels and 'dissolving tartarous humours' (*Pharmacopoeia* 480-1).

4 Corrected in MS from 75

have entred in my Booke but cannot [*find?*] your letter att present there remained then to Ballance due to me 64£-7s-0d, I thinke it apeares very plaine but if there bee any mistake I shall bee willing to rectifye it. As the old Account stands now in my Booke (distinct from these 2 last parcells) you will see by the inclosed account Current which hope you will prove satisfactory. This is the needfull att present from Sir   Yours etc.

Sent by the Sagamore Galley

69

London July: 28 1714

SIR

Above is Copy of what sent you by the Sagamore Galley. This comes by Capt Levered to informe you have sent you the Faecula Aronis, by this conveyance which I advised you I could not gett to send then; it will bee delivered you by by Mr William Rand your former man to whom I have sent some Medicines and therefore had the opportunity to putt it up with them. But the cheif designe of this to request another favour of you: you will see by the enclosed Bill of Loading for A case of Medicines for one Mr John Nicholls an Apothecary or Surgeon.[1] A person hee imployed here[2] to furnish him with an Invoyce hee sent him applyed himself to me who agreed with him on condition that as both hee that treated with me and Mr Nicholls were both altogether strangers to me that therefore I would consigne the goods to some freind. The sume they amount to is 43£ 6s 5½d sterling money (not New England money). Now his Freind here readyly consented they should bee soe consigned and upon his paying you the sayd sume, I intreat you, deliver them to him or, if hee bee a man of a good Character and substance as hee is represented to me to bee, deliver them however and let him pay the Freight and all charges you are att. I hope you'l excuse this trouble and in anything I can serve you as fair please to Comand it. I have sent him the invoyce and advised him to apply to you for them: hope the last things by Capt Corny arrived safe to you and prooved to your content. This att present is the needfull from etc.

1 John Nicholls, merchant and apothecary, seems to have been a substantial property owner in Boston as early as 1674. (See *First Report of the Record Commissioners of the City of Boston, 1876* [Boston 1876] 35, 38, 66, 80, 87, 96, 136, 150.) A John Nicholls of Boston was partner in three ships registered in Massachusetts 1706-8, with most of his partners being English (Masssachusetts Archives 7: 80, 335, 360). By 1714, he had been in the Artillery Company with Habijah Savage for twelve years and had held several minor town offices (Roberts *Military Company of Massachusetts* 1: 345).
2 Mr Cuttbeard; see below, letter 70.

70 TO MR JOHN NICHOLLS APOTHECARY ATT BOSTON IN NEW ENGLAND

July 28 1714

SIR

This comes with inclosed Invoyce for a Parcell of Druggs sent you by this Conveyance Capt Lithered. Your Freind Mr Cuttbeard treating with me about them wee att last agreed but as hee was altogether a stranger to me as well as yourself I agreed with him which hee willingly consented to that they should bee consigned to some Freind there who should have orders upon your satisfying for them to deliver them to you; according have consigned them to my Freind Mr Savage with whom I have dealt for 10 or 12 years and have sent him the Bill of Loading with directions to deliver them to you. The Character your Freind gives of you incourages me to bee ambitious of your correspondance and indeed it was cheifly the Expectation of farther dealings that made me comply with this parcell which being almost all Druggs there is very little gott by it. You see by the Invoyce have charged you with the Ensurance which was done with your Freinds consent for it was noe way reasonable for me to run the risque for soe very small advantage. The usuall way I trade with persons of your Country is at 65 perCent advance on the goods in New England money but have now agreed for this parcell to take Sterling money without advance. I have sent a smaller Quantity then you writ for of 2 or 3 things because of their extravagant prizes as Turmerick, Cortex Peru, etc but hope what is sent will bee sufficient to serve you till I heare from you againe. I have traded above 20 yeares to New England and am sure none can or will sell cheaper if as good, and therefore hope by next opportunity after you receive this to heare farther from you as your occasions require which shall Faithfully be remitted you. This is the needfull etc.

71 TO MR WILLIAM RAND[1] APOTHECARY ATT BOSTON IN NEW ENGLAND

July: 28 1714

SIR

Yours bearing date the 5 of May last I am favoured with Conteineing your Invoyce for Sundry Druggs and Medicines am willing to deale with you on

---

1 William Rand of Boston was born in 1689, son of Thomas and Sarah (Longley) Rand of Charlestown, Mass. He lost his father at the age of six, and was later an apprentice, or possibly a servant, of Habijah Savage. See above, letter 69. He married three times (Sarah Cotta, Isabella

the same terms as you propose vizt as Mr Savage dos and allways did which was cent per cent for what I bought out of my owne way with ready and 65 perCent for every thing else. But in your parcell there being nothing considerable (accept the Morters) out of my way I have made it all att 65 perCent advance and shall bee ambitious to settle a constant Correspondance with you where you may allways expect and shall [have] all the fayr and Candid usage you can desyre. I hope your Morter will please you; I tryed all about for a second hand Morter but could not gett one a farther [for: farthing?] cheaper than 9d a pound soe thought if I must give that price had better send a new one. I have sent everything you writt for accept the spicknard of which there is none to bee hade in London; it is worth 50s a pound and if you would give that price cant get it neither, but if you are in extreame want of it there is one Mr Thomas Barton of Salem in New England has some which I sent him some yeares ago and hee ment another thing, if hee has not disposed of it all I beleive hee will let you have half a pound of it. There is no difference between Lythurge of Gold and Silver[2] soe have sent the Quantity togather. Everything sent is good and charged very low being desyreous to encourage farther and larger dealings. Druggs generally are very Dear much Dearer then before the peace, the extravagant Duty layd on them ruines all. Cortex Peru is risen 75£ in a 100£ within this year and half: and Rad Curuma is 4 times the price it use to bee att. You shall allways bee supplyed as cheap as possible, this is the needfull etc. You will find a small parcell directed to Mr Savage which please to deliver to him.

Armitage, and Elizabeth Leeds), became a member of Old South Church in 1722, and joined the Artillery Company in 1732. A year later he was known to have an apothecary shop 'at the sign of the Unicorn, near the town dock.' Rand was also a practising physician who was in charge of the patients at the isolation hospital on Rainsford Island from 1737 to 1740. His notorious nephew and namesake, whom he helped finance through Harvard, served an apprenticeship with him before making his name as a rake and counterfeiter. William Rand senior died in Boston in 1758 (Roberts *Military Company of Massachusetts* 1: 451; Francisco Guerra *American Medical Bibliography, 1639-1783* [New York 1962] 467, 472, 545; Sibley *Harvard Graduates* 11: 163-4).

2 Litharge of gold and silver are lead salts produced in refining of the precious metals. Used on open wounds, they were regarded as generating flesh. They were also taken internally for diarrhoea, dysentery, and disorders of blood or urine (Salmon *Pharmacopoeia* 315; OED, s.v. 'Litharge').

72 MR ROBERT ANDERSON

Aug: 24 1714

SIR

Above is coppy of what I writ to you by Capt Lasselles Jan. 23 last[1] since which vizt June 12 last I writ you word of the unhappy losse of the said Capt Lassells who was castaway within a few days after hee sett sayle which was a very great losse and disapoytment for which I have been greatly concerned but could noe way avoyd it. For feare the want of the Medicines should prove to your farther disapoyntment I have by this conveyance the same Capt Lassells shipt you the same things againe as near as possible agreeing to the former Invoyce onely have sent but one pound of Cortex[2] now instead of 2 lbs before by reason it is growne soe extreame dear; inclosed is Invoyce and Bill of Loading of the same. You see I have taken off the advance on the last parcell and charged onely the prime cost because as a losse has happned I would make it as easye to you as possible. I have inclosed an Invoyce of the former parcell allsoe and to prevent any such losse againe I have ensured them soe that if any accident should fall out it shall not lye upon you which has been a conciderable charge to me. But I hope these will arrive safe to you and shall hope for and expect returns by the spring Shipps and wish I may then heare of your farther incouragement. This is the needfull but etc.   from   Sir Yours

JC

73 MR CONRADE ADAMS

Aug 24 1714

SIR

Above is Copy of what I writt you by Capt Lassells last voyage Since which vizt June 12 last I writt to you againe adviseing you of that misfortune that attended those things sent in Capt Lassells hee being cast away a few days after hee sayled from England and all was lost not a penny saved. Since which I have been favoured with severall from you with another Invoyce from Mr Phyllips much larger then the former allsoe a small one for your owne use and Another for Coll Browne all which I have put up and forwarded to you by this conveyance vizt Capt Lassells againe; wish him better

1 See above, letter 59.
2 *Cortex peru*

successe then before. I chose rather to send by him then another that if need bee hee might satisfye you of the misfortunes of the former Cargoe; these I have ensured soe if any damage come it will bee noe losse to any of the persons concerned. You will find all the parcells put up in one Case yours and Mr Brownes in 2 small Cases att the Bottom allsoe there is a small paper parcell directed for you with 2 or 3 things that your Case would not conteine which please to remember to ask Mr Phyllips for; you may easyly adjust the Freight with him which cannott bee much. The parcells were soe small I was afraid they would bee lost if they were putt up singly. I have taken off the advance from Mr. Phyllips parcell that was lost and have not charged the Ensurance for these that I have sent now to make him easye. You will receive letters by this conveyance from one Mr Suffeild who has sent you a Chest of Woolen Merchandize which I suppose hee has given you a perticuler account of; if hee meet with incouragement tis like hee will send more. I advised you in former letters that my Uncle Major Johnson is dead last March and that my sister has Administred on his estate; she was in hopes of receiving the Ballance of that account from you before now. If you have not sent it before this comes to hand please to hasten it for she wants it extreamely. I leave you to make returns in what you judge best onely if it bee in Sugar I intreat some of it may bee white. I request the Continuance of your Endeavours to procure more Invoyces. This is the needfull from Sir etc.

Advised him the reason of the rise of Pul v Chel o/g Comp.[1]

74 MR HABIJAH SAVAGE

London Dec: 4 1714

SIR

Take this opertunity per Man of Warr that is comeing expresse to you from the Government that I have received yours per Capt Spurryer and Capt Willard with the Loggwood, Silver and AmberGrease.[1] The Loggwood I have layd up for there is noe selling it without Cent per Cent losse tis not worth

---

1 *Pulvis è chelis cancrorum compositus*

1 Ambergris is a waxy substance secreted from the intestines of sperm whales. As it is found free-floating in the sea its identity was in doubt into JC's time. Josselyn thought it was a sea mushroom (*New England's Rarities* 36). Salmon valued it as 'a good Preservative against the Plague, and preserves the Spirits from infection' (*Pharmacopoeia* 355).

above 14-10 per Ton whether it may mend in the spring or not cannott tell. The Ambergrease I have not disposed off; it is but very ordinary, the Grey sort is best. Shall next opertunity advice farther about it. But there was surely a mistake about the Silver there not being full 48 ozs [?] and you charge 50s [*for: ozs?*]; I never had any before from you or any other person but what held out full weight. Hope if you inquire of the person you hade it off you may find out the mistake it was in noe persons hands but my owne and I am possitive there was noe more of it and I have given your Account Credit for noe more. There allsoe wanted ½ ounce of the Ambergrease but that might wast. Your small Invoyce I allsoe received but there has been noe ship gone since nor will not before February if there hade been any conveyance I would not have missed it; but by Capt Thomas who will bee the first Ship shall not fayle to send them and hope by that time may receive your generall Invoyce that I may send them both togather, if not I will send these. I thanke you for your care and trouble about Mr. Greaves money[2] to who if you see him pray give my service and accept the same yourself from Sir   Yours   JC

Att the same time and by the same conveyance writt allsoe to Mr John Nicholls adviceing him I purposed to send his Invoyce per next Shipping.

75 TO MR THOMAS GREAVES ATT CHARLES TOWNE NEW ENGLAND

London Mar: 15 1714/15

SIR

Yours per Capt Plaisted of November 7 last am favoured with, with a Small Invoyce inclosed, which I have putt up and this serves to cover Invoyce and Bill of loading for them in the Partridge Captaine Bond which I wish well to your hand and to your content. I understand by Mr Savage you have paid to him the former Ballance for which I returne you hearty thankes. I have carefully observed your letter, and taken perticuler care that every thing sent bee choice good. How the Cantharides[1] should prove bad I know not I am sure these are as new as any in Towne. Have put up the Sugar Candy in a Box to prevent any inconvenience. As to returnes if you can gett Bills of Exchange

---

2 See above, letters 66 and 68.

1 *Cantharides,* dried Spanish Fly, was used to raise blisters, as a diuretic, 'cleaner of the womb,' and aphrodisiac (Quincy, *Complete English Dispensatory,* 167-8, 229).

or[2] silver that dos best, I have frequently hade bills of exchange for a farr lesse sume then yours But if that cannott bee hade please to pay it as before to Mr Savage. As to what you write about oyles: as for oyle of Pennyroyall[3] it is worth very little there being very little of it used and in the drawing the water wee have more oyle comes off then wee have occasion for; for oyl of Gouldenrod[4] I never knew a drop of it used in my life nor doe I beleive there ever was a dram of it used in England; as for oyl of Mint if it bee the right Spearmint[5] it may sell for about 24s a pound, therefore if you thinke fitt to try a Quart Bottle of it first and when see what sort it is may judge better of it and if can give any incouragement shall bee glad to serve you in that or any other affayr and shall value myself by farther and greater dealings am Sir etc.   JC

76 TO MR JOHN NICOLLS ATT BOSTON IN NEW ENGLAND

London Mar: 17 1714/15

SIR

Yours of Sept. 19th 1714 I have received and take perticular notice of the contents and some complaints therein but hope upon second thought you will

2 'Nor' survived in the manuscript by oversight after Cruttenden changed 'if you cannot gett Bills of Exchange nor Silver you may ... ' to read as above.
3 A volatile oil obtained from the mint herb pennyroyal. It certainly had a place in the pharmacopoeias, even if it was not much used. Salmon valued the oil used internally or externally for relief of headache (*Pharmacopoeia* 84), perhaps a survival of an earlier belief that a garland of pennyroyal was effective against headache (Grieve *Modern Herbal* 2: 624-6). By the 1736 edition of Quincy the outward application for headache was still recommended, but the primary use of oil of pennyroyal was as an astringent, to promote menstrual flow or expulsion of the foetus, and it was also used in pleurisy, jaundice, and other disorders thought to arise from obstructions (*Complete English Dispensatory* 87). Edward Tuckerman notes that New England pennyroyal was a different variety than the English (*Transactions and Collections of the American Antiquarian Society* 4 [1860]: 175n).
4 The contemporary pharmacopoeias support Cruttenden with their silence on the virtues of oil of goldenrod. Greaves may have derived a medicinal use from earlier works like John Gerarde's famous *The Herbal* (1 vol. in 2 [London 1633] 1: 429-30), where goldenrod is valued as diuretic, melting and removing kidney stones and 'flegmatic humours,' as well as helping open wounds. Gerarde does not mention oil of goldenrod, and valued the herb in much the same way as Salmon valued a precipitate prepared from its roots. See faecula Aronis, above, letter 68, note 3.
5 Oil of mint could be oil of peppermint, spearmint, or pennyroyal, all fragrant volatile oils. Salmon valued oil of mint to warm and strengthen the stomach and prevent vomiting, which probably meant making medicines palatable (*Pharmacopoeia* 641). Subsequent to Cruttenden's time, peppermint became more valued medicinally than spearmint, see Grieve *Modern Herbal* 2: 533-6). Spearmint was successfully introduced into New England from old by settlers (Josselyn *New England's Rarities* 89).

find noe cause for it. I shall endeavour allways to use you as well as I can and I thinke I can doe it as well as any one else can. You cannot judge att such a distance of the rise or fall of Druggs many of which are now extravagant Dear. I have allsoe received your second Invoyce and by this conveyance have shipt them on the Partridge, Capt Bond which I wish well to your hand and to your content. I have taken the liberty you see which you gave me to alter the Quantitys of some things especially those were the Quantitys were very large as the Izinglasse Almonds[1] etc. or where they were extravagant dear.[2] Hope they will every way answear your expectation and you will have noe occasion of complaint which is very disagreable to me: and make noe doubt if you receive the Invoyce you mention from Mr Warner you will find mine cheapest. As for returnes I hade rather have it in Bills of Exchange or in peices of 8 if it can bee hade; as to what you desyre to know the price and custome of I have given you some account of in an inclosed paper by itself, Tho I beleive there is noe way soe good as by Bills of Exchange or in Spanish money. [*in margin*: price and duty Margarita[3] Rad Serpent[4] Castoris[5] Sperma Coeti.] You see by the Invoyce I leave you to your liberty to pay for them in Sterling money here or if in New England money att 65 perCent advance which is the custome of your Country to doe and which is much one to me

1 Isinglass is a whitish transparent gelatin derived from fresh water fish, especially sturgeon. Salmon notes that it 'is used in Gellies and Broths, with Sugarcandy: Of it is made Mouth Glew, which is sweet and glutinous; is good against Night-wheals, and serves to glew Instruments with, and seal Letters. It is reported to help the Lethargy; but I scarcely believe it' (*Pharmacopoeia* 214; OED; Josselyn *New England's Rarities* 32). Isinglass almonds could mean: isinglass, almonds; almonds coated with isinglass; or, most likely in this context, almond-shaped lumps of isinglass.
2 Crossed out: 'as Jallop etc. of which there is none to bee had att any price therefore have onely sent 2 lbs.'
3 Pearls. A ground pearl salt was used medicinally against a wide variety of pains, especially gout (Salmon *Pharmacopoeia* 382), though JC need not have been interested in making *spiritus Margaritarum* to be interested in importing pearls.
4 Use of two kinds of snakeroot, Virginia and Seneca (black), was borrowed from North American Indian medicine and they came to be valued as alexipharmic and as ingredients in plague water (Quincy *Complete English Dispensatory* 177; Healde *New Pharmacopoeia* 202). More extravagant claims for Seneca snakeroot were made by William Byrd (*The Prose Works*, ed. Louis B. Wright [Cambridge, Mass. 1966] 231, 272); and especially by Dr John Tennent (*Every Man His Own Doctor* [Williamsburg 1734]; *Essay on the Pleuresy* ... [Williamsburg 1736], and *An Epistle to Dr. Mead, concerning the epidemical Diseases of Virginia* ... [and] *the Seneca Rattlesnake Root* [Edinburgh 1738]). Although widely used in America in the later seventeenth century, and destined to become a major contribution to the pharmacopoeias of the next century, snakeroot was not introduced into England until the 1730s. Hence, in 1715, Cruttenden shows no interest in Nicholls' suggestion of it as a means of making returns, though he comments on each of his other suggestions later in this letter.
5 Castoris for castoreum; see above, letter 39, note 1.

onely would have you take notice that I will run noe risque and therefore have insured them out and I would advice you when you make returnes to give advice by some other Shipp that insurance may bee made time enough to prevent losse and damage as in the case of Capt Plasted who I hinted before to you was cast away but could not then tell whether the pearles you sent were lost or not; but I am now forced to send you the Melancholly news that they were for I spoke with Capt Plasted 2 days agoe (hee being but newly come to Towne) and he assured me they were lost being in the Chest where all his money was. Getting the Chest ashore a wave oversett the boat and soe they were lost but most of the goods remaineing in the Ship were saved; however of a bad providence it was well it was noe worse for hee tells me they were very small Baggs onely for a sample to try whether it would answeare or not which I am glad of. You mention nothing in your letter what the Quantity was: I have made the best in–[*in margins:* quiry I can about the Druggs you mention and find the duty soe extravagantly high I doe not thinke it will bee worth while to send them. Castor pays 3s 4d a pound duty and tis not worth above 5s beside losse on drying. Pearles are from 6s to 16s an ounce if fine orient; you may try a few first which may bee gott ashore without Entring, custome ruines all. If you cannott gett Bills or Spanish money you hade better send substantiall Comoditys as Loggwood, oyle, Turpentine or sugar which I have sometimes hade from your Country and which will turne to much better account. This is the needfull but Service etc. You must take care the Comoditys are not to deare.

77 TO MR CONRADE ADAMS

March: 14 1714[/*15*]

Yours under Care of Dr William Phyllips I received and by the same hands designed to have made the returnes but was prevented. I hope before this the Dr is arrived att his habitation in a better state of health then when hee left England which then was much better then when hee arrived here which was indeed very deplorable. While hee was here I shewed him all the civilitys I was capable off and assisted him in every thing I could and his money falling short I advanced for him about 40£. This I desyre your silence about if hee arive safe for then I doubt not but in honour hee will take care to repay mee; but if anything should intervene to hinder his safe arrivall I intreat your interest that I may bee reimbursed for I lent him the money and have his bond for it. I am in dayly expectations of returnes for Sister Bragge of the Ballance

of the account due to Major Johnson; allsoe of my owne returnes on Mr Phyllips and other accounts which I desyre may bee in sugars and if possible some
of them in first whites; allsoe hope for the Contenuance of your favours in
procureing as many Invoyces as possible which shall allways bee carefully forwarded to you; allsoe hope you will make returnes to Mr Brookes and Mr
Suffeild of what things they consigned to you. This is the needfull etc.

Sent in Capt Hankin

78 TO DR PHYLLIPS

London Mar: 15 1714/15

SIR

I heartyly wish this may meet you safely in Barbados and in a good state of
health which I shall greatly rejoyce to hear off. This is the first letter I have
writt since your departure hence I was glad to hear by yours to Mr Clutterbuck from Plymouth that you were soe much better but I cannot forbeare let-
ting you know that I tooke it a little unkindly that you should write to soe
manny and leave me out of the number. I never received one line from you
after I parted from you att Deptford I was told indeed that you charged me
with unkindnesse in that I denyed your request in sending you the last 6
pounds by your man. I cannot tell what message he might bring you but I am
sure I delivered none to him that you had any reason to take amisse you knew
very well I severall times asked you what money you should have occasion for
and the most you ever told me was 30£ which you hade and att last when you
rose to 6 or 7 more you still hade it and if you hade desyred more then you
should have hade it but after the matter was settled and the Bond made there
must have been the charges of a new Bond and, which was more to me att
that time, I must have made another Journey to Deptford which in the hurry
I then was would have been very troublesome to me; and besides not in the
least expecting you would have any farther occasion I hade not 6£ in the
house when your man came. I am afraid this was not the onely instance
wherein your best freinds were misrepresented and those who were onely pretended ones incouraged. However it bee I have the satisfaction I advised you
for the best as farr as I was able and tho it was chargeable to you as it was I
am confident if you hade lodged all the time att Millers the charge would
have been double. Haveing thus eased my mind I declare my resolution to re-
taine an inviolable Freindship on my part and shall bee allways ready to
serve you upon all occasions wherein I am capable and please myself with the

prospect of continueing a yearly Correspondance with you by letters and traffick. Shall bee glad if you could recommend me to any responsible Chaps.[1] Desyre returnes may bee made in white Sugar. This with service is the needfull etc.

[*in margin:* Sent in Capt Hankin]

79 TO MR THOMAS BARTON OF SALEM IN NEW ENGLAND

London Mar: 1714/15

SIR

Yours of Nov 27 last I am favoured with with Invoyce inclosed which I have complyed with and this incloses Invoyce and bill of loading of the same in the Partridge Capt Bond which I wish well to your hands and to your content which I have endeavoured to the uttmost of my power. I have carefully observed your directions and every thing in your Invoyce is sent onely the Turbith which is not to bee hade which I have severall times advised you off I have not heard of any hath been brought in this 20 yeares. Wee use to make use of Jallop for it but can't doe that now that being 12s a pound and noe Quantity to bee hade for that neither which is the reason I have sent but 2 lbs instead of 6 lbs and that is in powder to, being some powdered before the rise of it but is the true sort and very good. I was forced to doe the same by others, a man may goe to 20 Shops and not gett a pound of it. I like your proposall well of makeing returnes in Silver if it can bee hade for there is lesse trouble in it tho if you send it would bee glade to have advice of it by some other Ship for tho there is peace yet there is still great Hazzard. Capt Plumsted[1] by whom your letter came was cast away near home and all his money on board lost tho his Loggwood etc was saved and your letter that came by him was sopt in Saltwater that it was scarce legible and allmost tore to peices. I hade 2 Baggs of pearle in her which was lost. I have observed what you write about white Sugar but it is vastly risen since you were here and 20 perCent dearer this year then any before; however I have sent you 1 cwt of Loaves[2] which cost me every farthing 4£ 4s and were I to buy a Ton of it could not buy it a farthing cheaper. I have put it in with the same advance as the rest. I hope

---

1 Chapmen, pedlars, merchants or customers (OED; Tucker *Protean Shape* 264)

1 JC called him Plasted, letter 76.
2 Presumably loaf sugar

the Labell papers are such as you mean, desyre you will allways bee as perticuler as you can in every thinge. This is the need full etc.

[*in margin*: By the same Conveyance Capt Bond writ to Mr George Jackson
pressing him to make returns this year and to Mr John Emerson desyreing
him to use his interst with Mr Jackson to comply therewith.]

80 TO MR WILLIAM RAND

London Mar: 22 1714/15

SIR

Yours of October 28 last I am favoured with and was not a little concerned
att the contents thereof but doubt not you have found out Your mistake; the
Liquids you mention were certainely sent with the other things and suppose
putt up in a small Case or Box which was put into the outward great Case
and soe att your first opening them you might not bee apraised of it. I am
very possitive they were put up and Suppose the case not being full The violls
and Gally potts were added to fill up the vacancys which was the reason of
their omission. I doubt not before this comes to hand you will have found out
where the mistake was for I have hade a great deale of concerne about it But
am possitive they were sent. Hope by the first opertunity to receive a full satisfaction from you that they are received and wish may att the same time receive a further order from you which I shall very readly comply with being
very willing to keepe up a constant Correspondance with you and shall allways take perticular care to furnish you with what is good and as cheap as
possible. I hope you were soe kind as to deliver the small parcell I desyred you
to give to Mr Habijah Savage haveing not yet been favoured with any advice
from him that hee hade received it. This is the need full but tenders of hearty
service etc.

81 MR HABIJAH SAVAGE

Mar 18 1714/15

SIR

I have received severall letters from you this fall the contents of which I carefully observe as allsoe your Invoyce which I have forwarded to you by this
conveyance The Partridge, Capt Bond. I sometime since advised you I designed to Ship them in Capt Thomas which I fully intended but att last hee

disapoynted me and could not take them in. This is an extraordinary good ship, and hope may arrive there near as soon as the other. Inclosed is Invoyce and Bill of loading of the same which I wish well to you and every way to your intrye satisfaction. I have noted your complaints of overchargeing and could wish you were here yourself and then you would bee fully satisfyed that if you hade with your ready money bought this parcell now sent you would not have saved 5£ perCent. As for Drugs I am sure I can buy them as cheap as any one and for the Colours I tryed about att severall shops and where I could buy them cheapest I hade them and paid ready money for them. I wish you hade been more perticuler as to the painting there being severall sorts of allmost every thing you write for there is of the Smalt[1] sorts from 6d to 4s a pound. I consulted the likely persons I could about it and they advised me to this sort which I have sent att 10d per lb which they assure me will answeare any use you have to putt it to. But if you would write whether you would have the first, second, or third sort I could then bee more exact for if possible I would comply with your orders exactly. I have inclosed the state of your account from the beginning of our Correspondance which is as exact as I can compute it and hope it will exactly agree with yours and prove Satisfactory. Please to observe the 2 first parcells I sent you amounting to 433-14-6 is Ballanced by by receipts from you in May 1709 and Aprill 1710 by severall Comoditys not all perticulerly mentioned in my Booke amounting to 369-7-6 soe that there then remained to Ballance 74£ 7s. Since which time I have expressely mentioned by whom and what every sume remitted has been and shall continue to doe soe constantly for the future. By this account it appeares that your dealing has been very conciderable and your payments extraordinary good and I wish I were able to expresse myself soe as to satisfye you fully how much I price and value your custome and I am sure any jealousy of looseing it would be very uneasy to me especially if I were conscious to myself of haveing done anything to deserve it. Therefore if possible I would once for all let you know that if I can cleare but 10 perCent I will not loose your Custome; but to make a just estimate of profitt on trade you must dully consider the vast losse upon every thing returned. The last returnes you made in Capt Willard amounted to 247-2-6 and before I gott the Loggwood into the warehouse instood[2] me in about 125£ Sterling more which 2 sumes make 372-2-6 and I have not sold the Loggwood yet nor cannot make of it and your Ambergrease above 215£. Now if you compute the losse of this you will finde the

---

1 Smalt is a pigment made by pulverising glass coloured blue with cobalt (OED).
2 'Instood' not in OED. The MS cannot possibly read 'it stood,' though that presumably conveys the meaning.

profit very small and beside you may observe I make noe distinction in the
advance of those things bought with ready money out of my owne way then of
the Medicines whereas you know you formerly allowed Cent perCent for
what was out of my owne way and bought with ready money. This I hope is
sufficient to satisfye you how desyreous I am to continue your Freindship and
dealing. As to what you mention of one Hawkins sending soe much cheaper I
can onely say hee must bee lead into some mistake or other or else expects to
[*be?*] paid for them here in Sterling money for I know the man and deale conciderably with him myself and have sold him a great many things this last
year and am sure hee cannott afford them cheaper then I doe nor will not
when hee finds the losse soe great upon returnes. You'l observe in the account
of the Bills you sent me that I adde the Advance you gave for them and not
the Sterling money. I take notice of what you observe of the Lockyers Pills[3]
and am possitively sure they were not of the right sort haveing never bought
them for any such price. I have read your letter to the person I bought them
of and hee asserts hee never sold them to anyone cheaper then hee did to me
and I doe not know why hee should for I paid him emediately for them. I
know they may bee bought soe about the Towne but then they are not made
by the first proprietors and if you are contented with those will send you what
you will att the same price but you desyred to have them true. And I remember once above 20 yeares agoe I sent over by order 100 boxes of them to one
Mr Cooper of your Towne[4] and hee sent them back againe in great Anger
and I lost a great deale by them soe that in your next please to signifye which
sort you will have for there are severall here that pretend to make them and
for any thing I know they may bee as good. And as for your Complaint of the
Galls[5] they were then att that price and if you hade been here you could not

3 Cotton Mather, in his unpublished work 'The Angel of Bethesda,' written between 1720 and
1724, did not like Lockyer's pills, though he favoured a regular vomit for health and the pills
were for that purpose. Mather quoted approvingly 'an eminent Physician' as follows: 'It is well
known (he says), that a pretended Chymist, who calls himself Lockyer, hath gained by a Pill
many thousand Pounds, which is one of the vilest and most contemptible among all the mineral
Praeparations I ever yett knew tried in Medicine' (printed in Otho T. Beall and R.H. Shryock
Cotton Mather, First Significant Figure in American Medicine [Baltimore 1954] 223). Lockyer's pills
were still being advertised for sale in the American colonies in the last third of the century
(Young and Griffenhagen 'Old English Patent Medicines' 717).
4 Thomas Cooper is the only taxable of that name on Boston's list for 1695 (Nathaniel Dearborn
Boston Notions [Boston 1848] 271; *Report of Boston Record Commissioners* 22, 23, 106, 139, 152, 160).
5 Salmon considered the galls of animals as having cutting and purgative qualities and as curing
certain eye and ear diseases. He noted that of animals bulls' gall was most effective and of birds
that of partridge. The galls could be used as waters, extracts, or tinctures, 'but the most famous is
the Tincture or Fucus of Ox Gall' (*Pharmacopoeia* 238-9).

have bought them cheaper but they rise and fall 2 or 3 times in a year. Jallop
now is worth 12s a pound I cannot buy it for a farthing lesse nor for that neither any quantity, for there is none of it to bee hade; now you cannott bee
sensible of this att such a distance but are ready to thinke I impose upon you,
I have therefore sent but 3 lbs. I hope it will bee cheaper ere long. You see I
have charged you but half as much for the Turmerick as I did before because it
is cheaper, and depend upon it you shall allways have the Advantage of the fall
of the Markett. I thinke the volatile Spiritts are as pungent as can bee made. I
Beg your pardon for what I writ to Mr Nicolls I designed noe hurt in it and depend on it I shall never bee guilty of such a thing againe. I have you see allowed for the Breakage in your account. Capt Plasted by whom your letters
came was cast away and the letters lay some time in Salt water that when they
came to hand they were rot to peices and scarce legible soe that if you hade not
sent a Duplicate by another Conveyance should have been att a great losse. I
mention this to suggest how necessary it is [to] write by more then one Conveyance. I have given your account Credit but for 48 [ozs ?] of plate in the last parcell for as I suggested to you in a former letter there was noe more and I hope
you are satisfyed and have found out the mistake. I cannot gett off the Ambergrease tis the Black sort and the Grey sort (that is marbled like the inside of a
Nuttmegg) is the most valuable tho noe sort sells well now for it is very much
growne out of use.[6] I am afraid I shall not make 12s an ounce of it I can buy the
fine Grey sort of it for 24s. As for returnes if can bee hade desyre may be in
Plate or Bills of Exchange but if cannott bee hade must leave it to your prudent
management if you should sent Loggwood you must not give deare for it there
for tis exceedingly low here. This is the need full but etc.

82 TO MR JAMES HENDERSON ATT NEW YORKE

London Apr: 6 1715

SIR

I am favoured with both your letters and take notice of your complaint of
Damage etc. in the first but hope upon Examination it did not apeare soe
great as it seemed att first. By your order in the second letter of 3 Sept I have
sent you the Small parcell following viz etc. They come in the William, Capt
Dove and inclosed is a receipt for their comeing on board and a promise from

6 Salmon, in the edition of his *Pharmacopoeia* printed in the following year, shows no such waning
enthusiasm (355).

the Captaine to deliver them to you free of charges upon your producing that note. I did it to prevent charges as much as I could there being a Tax on Bills of loading.[1] I hope they will come safe to you; I have paid the Freight and all charges. The Chamomell Flowers[2] were not in your order but your Freind called on me and ordered me to send them. You see there is but 1 lb of Jallop instead of 6 lbs; the reason is it is soe exceeding dear and Scarce; tis worth 12s a pound for me to buy and cannot gett any quantity for that neither; I hade a small quantity ground for makeing Rozen by me before it grew soe very dear which is the reason have sent it in powder. I hade orders from severall att New England for large quantitys of it but could onely send 2 or 3 lbs instead of 15 or 20; wee hope to have some arrive ere long. By your Freind I have received the 2 Jarrs of what you call Sperma Coeti but have not received above a weeke; whether you hade justice done or not I cannot tell but neither of the Jarrs were above one third part full, there was in both but 9 pounds. I am afraid shall bee able to make very little or nothing of it for I never saw any thing like it; I have hade severall times unrefined Sperma Coeti from New England but then it has been of a solid body dry tho not white which use to gett refined allowing one half for doing it, but this is perfectly liquid, seemes to bee nothing but Traine oyle.[3] However I will consult the refiner and make the most I can of it and give you Credit for it. Would have sent by Capt Tucker but he could not take it. Shall bee glad of farther Correspondance etc the needfull etc.

83 MR THOMAS BARTON

London Aug: 22 1715

SIR

Yours of Feb. 17 and allsoe of June 14 are both under veiw the Contents of both which I take notice of. I hade procured your Alembick, wormetub[1] and

---

1 This seems to be Cruttenden's first recorded concern for an act in force since 1711 (9 Anne c. 23 *Statutes* 12: 242). His practice of sending small packages as a single shipment saved this tax. See below, letter 122.

2 Camomile is a medicinal herb considered a mild carminative, discussant, and purgative. A decoction of the flowers in Rhine wine was valued to settle the stomach, but primarily as a specific for stones and gravel (Salmon *Pharmacopoeia* 39-40; Short *Medicina Britannica* 41-2).

3 Whale oil

1 Alembic and wormtube were distillation equipment.

Sand[2] before the arrivall of your last letters; hade a little roome left in the worme Tubb which I filled up with part of new Invoyce of which part and all the old Invoyce this Incloses a Coppy of, and Bill of Loading Shipt in Capt Thomas in the Amity, which I wish well to your hands and to your Content. The remaining part shall (if please God)[3] bee shipt you by Capt Savage who will sayl in a Month att furthest. Capt Thomas being ready to sayle within a few days after your letters came was the occasion I could not send you the whole but hope you will shortly receive them. Your 140 ozs Silver by man of warr is not yet come to hand but hope to receive it in a few days; I thanke you for your care therein and am not uneasye about your being soe much in my debt but if you hade goods to your satisfaction could bee glad it was more. Jallop continues still very Dear those that I deale with att Boston I am forced to send them not above a Quarter of what they write for. I know a Gentlemen paid ready money 11s a pound a few days agoe for a Quantity of it; wee are in hopes it will fall but feare it will never come to its old price againe by reason of the extravagant duty on it and on all Druggs which is a very great discouragement on all trade. Every thing in your first order is sent accept the Jujubes[4] and Sebestens[5] which cannott bee gott wee allways use Raysins for them which to bee sure are as good I have not seen one of them this 7 years. I hope you'l like the Alembick and worm; I beleive tis cheaper then a second hand one for them tis impossible to know their wear. The founders sand[6] is in the Cask, it cost me every farthing 5s a Bushell. I can't yet give you any account of your Bill of 6£ 4s whether it will bee accepted and paid or not, haveing yet hade noe advice from my Freind about but hope shall bee able to advice you per Capt Savage as allsoe of the receipt of your money per the Phoenix man of warr. This is the needfull att present etc.

[*in margin:* Note to inquire after his Kinsman, and advise by Savage]

2 Founder's sand; see below, note 6.
3 Closing parenthesis added
4 'They are a long Fruit, almost like an Olive, with one Stone, and taste like a Raisin; they grow in Italy upon the Ziziph tree. They are pectoral, good against Coughs, Colds, Hoarseness, Pleurises, spitting of Blood, Sharpness of Urine, and Corrosion of Reins and Bladder' (Salmon *Pharmacopoeia* 120).
5 A prune-like fruit of Middle Eastern *Cordiu Myxa,* valued against catarrhs, constipation and fevers (*ibid.* 125; OED).
6 Fine sand with a small clay content which facilitates its being moulded for casting.

84 MR HABIJAH SAVAGE

London Aug 22 1715

SIR

Yours per Captaine Thornton and Capt Combs with the Loggwood in each are come safe I was surprised att the mistake in the first but was glad to find your were sensible of it and hade rectifyed it in the second. Your Invoyce by Combs comeing to hand but a few days agoe it was impossible I should compleat your Invoyce to send by this Conveyance but I purpose to send them [by] your Brother Capt Savage who is putt up for Boston and will sayle he tells me in 3 weekes times by whom you may expect your order. I am sorry you sent Loggwood; there is nothing worse can bee sent; tis not worth here above 11£ 5s or 11£ 10s att most. What you sent by Capt Willard last year I have still by me[1] which with the charges of these now sent amount to above 400£ and if I sell it now cannot make half that sume of it, and when or whether ever it bee any better I cannot tell. However it cannott bee helped soe must doe as well as I can with it, tho tis a hard article to have soe much money lye dead I intreat you will bee very cautious in sending any more. If upon inquiry I am able to give advice what to make returnes in shall doe it by next conveyance. This is the Needfull etc.

85 MR JOHN NICOLLS

London Aug: 22 1715

SIR

Yours of March 9 per Capt Parnell as allsoe yours of May 12 per Capt Hutton with the Silver in each and the Cortex Wint[1] and yours of July 6 by the Phoenix with advice of the Pitch and Rice in Capt Mangier which is not yett arrived. [in margin: ozs 34½, ozs 18½, Silver: 1-8, Cortex Wint 1 cwt] The Contents of all which letters I note and your Invoyce I have complyed with and have sent by this conveyance Capt Thomas in the Amyty Invoyce and

---

1 See above, letter 81.

1 *Cortex winteranus,* or Winter's bark, is from an evergreen of the magnolia family native to the South American highlands. It was named for Sir William Winter, the Elizabethan admiral who first recognized its antiscorbutic value. In 1693 Hans Sloane denounced the widespread substitution of Jamacian pepper tree bark for Winter's bark in London apothecary shops (Brooks *Sir Hans Sloane* 101-3; Salmon *Pharmacopoeia* 20).

bill of Loading of which comes inclosed. I wish them well to your hand and to your Content. I have sent every thing you writ for accept the Rad Contrayerva which is not to bee gott. I have varyed a little in the Quantitys of some things that are extreame deare as Jollop, Assafielda,[2] Nuttmeggs,[3] and oyl of Cinnamon[4] which are extravagantly dear but for the most part have sent the just Quantity you writt for. I was att a great losse what you ment by Pix Graeca.[5] I have made all the inquiry I can but cannot gett satisfaction in it some say tis comen Ship pitch (which wee allways use for it in makeing Basilicon[6] which is the onely medicine that I know off wherein it is prescribed) others say tis Colophy or Black Rozin[7] but I thought these you have in plenty soe could not intend them; have therefore sent you A bladder of Burgundy pitch which suppose will be usefull to you tho it bee not what you mean, pray in your next be more exact about it. You will find printed directions putt up in the Chest for the Spirit Cockl purg.[8] The Chest was not large enough to hold all soe have sent the Sweet Fennell[9] seeds in a double Bag which hope will come as safe. As to the Cupping Engine,[10] there is 2 ways of

2 *Asafoetida*, or Devil's dung, a resinous gum of strong garlic odour obtained from a Central Asian plant. Its medicinal value derived from its earlier use as an amulet against communicable diseases which, as Bauer notes (*Potions, Medicines* 16, 48-9), was probably effective because its smell would discourage close contact. Salmon valued it chiefly for disorders of the spleen and suffocation of the womb, and to heal open wounds (*Pharmacopoeia* 139).

3 Used as a stimulant, tonic, and alexipharmic. Nutmeg's effects on the brain were also recognized indirectly (Salmon *Pharmacopoeia* 19; Bauer *Potions, Medicines* 224-5; Grieve *Modern Herbal* 2: 591-2).

4 The fragrant oil of cinnamon, 'one of the greatest vegetable cordials,' was valued against colds, consumption, and conditions caused by dampness and was said to fight plague, poisons, fevers, and venemous bites (Salmon *Pharmacopoeia* 413-14).

5 See below, note 7.

6 Basilicon is a medicinal ointment.

7 Colophony or black rosin, formerly called 'Greek pitch' (OED), was derived from distilling common turpentine. The rosin was boiled in drinks to fight remains of venereal disease, to induce coughing, or to cleanse the urinary tract (Quincy *Complete English Dispensatory* 131).

8 Spirit of cockle purge, a decoction of the herb cockle valued for breaking and expelling stones, fighting serpent bites and the plague, and cleansing and healing old wounds (Salmon *Pharmacopoeia* 73).

9 Seeds of sweet or Roman fennel were used in fennel water and in gripe water to settle stomach, ease flatulence, and allay griping (Grieve *Modern Herbal* 1: 293-7). Josselyn noted that in New England fennel had to be potted in the autumn and kept indoors all winter (*New England Rarities* 90).

10 Cupping was a method of drawing blood away from an inflammation. A glass cup is applied firmly to dry skin nearby. A partial vacuum, created by heating the air in the glass before application or by use of pump, draws the blood within the circumference of the glass rim. In some cases it would then be drawn off through small wounds (*Ency. Brit.* 7: 635). The cupping engine was rather new at this time, as can be seen from Claver Morris *The Diary of a West-Country Physician* ed. Edmund Hobhouse (London 1934) 71.

useing them one with a Pump and another sort of glasses to bee used without fire but a sett of them glasses and the Pump would cost more than the Engine.[11] The Engine serves indifferently for both and may as well bee used with these comon glasses as with them soe that if you desyre to have the other sort you may send againe next time. Dr Davis which is lately come to your place has a sett of them which I suppose you may see. The Cortex Wintera-nus is not worth the Custome it cost. Most of your Invoyces being Druggs (and very few Medicines) upon which is very little and upon manny of them noe profitt att all but bought with ready money; the 65 perCent is to little and reckoning the extreme losse upon all returnes is scarce worth the trouble and therefore you must not expect I should recede from my first agreement that the risque shall not lye upon me; therefore I have as before ensured on these goods and charged the ensurance. If you concider the prodigious losse upon returnes you must owne this very reasonable. Other persons that send any other sort of goods sell them for 150 perCent advance And I can see noe reason why they should have soe much more advance then wee in our busy-nesse when things are bought well and Charged the prime Cost. I hope this may suffice to satisfye you that all may have noe farther dispute with you which is noe way gratefull to me.[12] Depend on it you shall have all the Can-dour and faithfullnesse you can expect in any dealing with me; you know att first I left you to your choice whether to pay me here in Sterling Money with-out advance or att 65 perCent advance and make returnes in your money. I desyre in your next you'l signifye which you choose that I may make your ac-count Debit and Credit accordingly. Allsoe I desyre if you send any more money you'l be carefull in lookeing it over for there was one piece as brasse as a Kettle which I cannot make a farthing off. This is the needfull etc.

86

Aug 25 1715

I writt a large letter to Mr Thomas Perkins Adviceing him I had sent over a power of Attourney to Mr Crawford and Poyntz Merchants in Kingston to sue him and to recover by law (unlesse hee doe it without) The 200£ Sterling which hee owned he had sold my goods for to Dr Tredway: which power I

11 The 'engine' referred to here might be a 'scarificator,' a spring-run device with numerous sharp cutting wheels used to make as many shallow incisions prior to cupping (OED, s.v. 'scarificator').
12 In the now obsolete sense of pleasing, acceptable, or welcome (OED)

sent by Mr William Arbuckle (who was one of the 3 wittnesses to it) to the above sayd Gentleman in a letter to them with perticuler information of the whole transaction between Mr Perkins and myself and Instructions how to proceed against him and how to make returnes when they hade received the money and promised to repay what charges they were to Mr Freenly here (who advised me to employ them) or to any other person they should appoynt and presed them to forward the matter with all expedition.

87 TO DR NATHANIEL LUCAS ATT BARBADOS

London Oct: 18: 1715

SIR

Your Invoyce under favour of Mr Conrade Adams came safe to hand which I have forwarded to you by this Conveyance Capt Lassells, wish [for: which] I wish safe to your hands and that they may prove entyrely to your Content and satisfaction. I have packt them in 2 cases the Dry and the liquid each by themselves that if any bottle should give way noe damage may accrew to the dry things; I have taken all possible care in the package and hope their will bee nothing broke tho after all the care possible sometimes through the rough usage on board Ship in stowing an accident may happen. I thought myself obliged to write perticulerly to you to inform you that I shall bee glad to settle a constant correspondance with you and to assure you I shall bee allways ambitious to serve you and promise you shall find all the Candid dealing you can desyre or expect. I have sent every thing of the best and charged the price as low as possible tho the advance bee lesse then I ever sent any in my life yet haveing hade very conciderable dealing with Mr Conrade Adams and with his Brother William before am willing still to try tho there bee very little prospect of advantage; tis very rare that there is any returnes made but there is as much losse as the advance of these goods amounts to. Hope this will bee but the begining of farther and greater dealings with you. The new duty of 20 perCent on all Druggs is a very discouragement to trade and renders all Druggs very dear. This is the needful but tenders of hearty service etc.   JC

88 DR FRANC JEMMETT

London Oct: 18 1715

SIR

Your Invoyce under favour of Mr Conrade Adams is come safe to hand which I putt up and forwarded to you by this Conveyance Capt Lassells which I wish well to your hand, and hope they will prove entyrely to your Satisfaction. I have packt them as you directed the Dry things in a strong Chest the Liquids by themselves and both soe carefully packt that I thinke tis impossible any manner of damage can come. I thought myself obliged to write to you to informe you how ambitious I am and shall allways bee to serve you and hope for the future there will never bee any cause of complaint. You complained of the Diapente[1] as not good the last time; it was such as the Grinders sell but that it may intyrely answeare your expectation I have done what I never did before in my life have beat it att home soe that there is the full proportion of every thing and as good as if it were to bee taken by the best Nobleman. I dare affirme there is not such a quantity of Diapende soe good in Europe; that you might not thinke the price to great have in the Margent sett downe the prime cost of each Ingredient.

[*in margin:* 21 Birthwort roots[2]   1-8-0
          21 Myrrh   5-5-0
          21 BayBerrys[3]   0-7-0
          21 Ivory   0-7-0
          21 Gentian[4]   0-13-0
             Beating   0-15-0
                     8-15-0]

I doe assure you I would not have had the trouble for any one else but to oblige you. I am sure you will find one pound goe farther then 3 pound of any can bee bought and that ordinary stuff I cannot now buy under 12d a pound

---

1 Diapente is an alexipharmic of ancient usage. Cruttenden's list of ingredients (above) in equal parts conforms to the recipe; without the ivory shavings it was known as a diatessaron (Frank P. Foster *An Illustrated Encylopedic Medical Dictionary* 3 vols. [New York 1888-90] 2: 1299; Robert Hooper *Medical Dictionary* 7th ed. [London 1839] 516). Diapente is not mentioned in Culpeper *English Physician*, Salmon *Pharmacopoeia*, or Quincy *Complete English Dispensatory*.

2 Salmon considered that this herbal root of temperate Europe and Asia, when mixed with a little myrrh, was a good laxative, and would bring on birth and afterbirth (*Pharmacopoeia* 2). Also see Grieve *Modern Herbal* 1.104.

3 Bayberry plaster, husked bayberries plus a multitude of added ingredients, is the only medicinal use of bayberry noted by Salmon. The plaster was to expel wind or alleviate pain in the head, stomach, liver, spleen, womb, or bowels (*Pharmacopoeia* 680).

4 Root of a common European herb, valued as a purgative and antidote to poison. As a purgative it was considered useful in a wide variety of complaints, and was expected to kill worms and expel birth and afterbirth (*ibid.* 9).

by reason Myrrh[5] is soe extreame dear. That Myrrh I made it with cannott bee bought for 3 times the price it use to bee, and indeed the new duty of 20 perCent layd on all Druggs is a very great discouragement to trade. This I am sure if you hade been here yourself you could not have bought with ready money this parcell of goods sent you for the price I charge them, soe willing I am to settle a constant correspondance with you. I am with humble Service Yours etc.   JC

89 DR WILLIAM PHYLLIPS

London Oct: 18 1715

SIR

Yours beareing date July 12 last I have received with the inclosed Bill for fourty four pounds on Messiers Rowland and William Tryon which Bill I have received and have here inclosed sent you back the Bond Cancelled; and for the 6s 5d which the Bill was more then the Bond I have sent you 9 Lancetts[1] which cost me the same sume, soe that we are even on that account. And as to that part of your letter that mentions my chargeing you with not writeing to me when you did to others wherein you say you writ to noe person after you went on board att Deptford till you came to Barbados all I can say is I saw a letter subscribed with your name to it dated from Plymouth to Mr Clutterbuck and another to the Musicioner that lodged there but there is an end of that. As to what Messages your man might bring you I can not help but I doe possitively assert I never spoke a word to him in all my life about any such thing as if I questioned how I should bee repayd againe. But if hee brought you such messages it would have been more Freindly in you to have told me of it that I might have vindicated myself rather then to take offence before you knew there was any ground for it. I am informed by Mr Adams that you hade taken a prejudice against me and hade settled a Correspondance with another Apothecary when you were in London and that you would have noe farther dealing with me. If this bee true I can't but take it very unkindly att your hands, and must say I thinke all things concidered I deserved better treatment from you. But if you are fixt with any other I shall bee easy

5 Myrrh, a gum resin from Middle Eastern balsam, was used as a purgative, and for chest ailments; tincture of myrrh was used in ointments for dressing wounds (Quincy *Complete English Dispensatory* 317-18; Salmon *Pharmacopoeia* 148-9; J.J. Keevil et al. *Medicine and the Navy* 4 vols. [London 1957-63] 2: 158).

1 A lancet is a surgical instrument with a double-edged blade, used for lancing boils, abscesses, etc.

about it being satisfyed with my owne integrity in every thing I did and I doubt not but, in lesse than 7 yeares you find as much and more cause to change againe then ever you hade from me. If there have been any misunderstanding between Mr Adams and you tis hard I must suffere by it. But after all I doe not find by your letter but that you have thought of farther Correspondance if soe all I can say is I shall be very glad to serve you, and promise nothing shall bee wanting on my part to keepe the Freindship intyre. I could have been glad to have heard your recovery hade been more compleat but rejoyce to heare tis soe well, and wish this may find your health more confirmed. Your freindship in recommending any practioners to me shall bee ever kindly accepted. This is the needfull but hearty wishes for your health and wellfare I remained etc.   JC

90 MR CONRADE ADAMS AND COMPANY

Lond Oct: 18 1715

SIR

Yours beareing Date July 4th last is come safe to hand with Invoyce and Bill loading for 4 hoggsheads and 2 Teares Sugar per Capt Harris which safe and well (as did allsoe those to Mr Suffeild and Brookes) for which give you hearty thankes; one of the Tearess which you call third white was very little if att all better then the hoggsheads and I did not sell it for a farthing more then they. Allsoe Inclosed came your Invoyces for self, Dr Lucas and Dr Jemett all which I have putt up and forwarded by this conveyance Capt Lassells, hope they will all prove to your and their satisfaction, I have done all in my power that they may doe soe. Have writ to each of them and inclosed which please to deliver them with the goods; allsoe inclosed is the Key of Mr Jemmetts Chest. I have shewed Sister Bragge what you writ relateing to her affayr and she has been with a Publick Notary with A Copy of the Letter of Admmistration she had taken out on Major Johnsons Estate and the Notary assures her that there is noe manner of occasion to goe before the Lord Major as you mention and gett the City seale to it which will cost near 20s but he has taken a Copy of the Administration which is here inclosed which hee says is as full a power as you can have and what hee has done 20 times in the same case. She is ruined by the Major hee oweing her Eleven hundred pound and noe person but she has or can have any claime to a farthing till she is payd and all he left her, if the debts can bee gott in, will not pay her half her debt. Her circumstances are soe streight she cant afford to lay out 20s and if she did it would not bee any more security to you. If you are not satisfyd will engage to indempnifye you from any damage, for I myself tooke out the letters for her of Administration and therefore I begg you will not put her off any farther but returne the Ballance of her account by the first spring Shipps for she is in very great nessessity of it. I am forced to advance money for her till it comes. As for returnes for these goods I desyre you will act as for yourself and let it bee with as much speed as you can and, if you can, lett there bee att least one Cask of white Sugar which serves for my owne use. Your freindship in procureing what Invoyces you can will allways bee thankfully owned by Sir   Yours etc.

91 MR GEORGE STEWART OF BOSTON IN NEW ENGLAND

London Feb: 18 1715/16

SIR

Pursant to your advice and order of July 5th last inclosed conteins Invoyce and Bill of Loading for a Parcell of goods Shipt on board the Province Gally, Capt Arthur Savage which wish well to your hands and hope they will prove intyrely to your content and satisfaction and hope may prove a begining of a farther correspondance and greater dealing. The case not being quite full have put up half a Grosse of Gallypotts which I supose cannott bee unusefull to you. I have sent pretty near the Quantity of every thing accept the Saffron of which you write for 2 lbs and have sent but one because I doubt whether you concidered the price it being a riseing Comodity and like to bee very dear; wee haveing hade the severest winter that has been for above 30 yeares which has very much destroyed the Saffron tis likely it may bee double the price next year; however you will have opertunity of sending advice frequently and att any time you shall have your orders complyed with onely must desyre you allways to bee as perticuler as you can as in your Morter you should have given advice near what weight you would have hade it. I have charged you the same advance as I doe other people but desyre your returnes may bee in Bill of Exchange or Silver if you can for there is such vast losse upon allmost all sort of goods that tis greater then the advance upon the goods outward. This is the needfull att present but hearty service etc.

92 MR THOMAS BARTON

London Feb: 18 1715/16

SIR

Yours of Aug. 4 last past have received with the 175 ounces of Silver have received safe with your additionall Invoyce which I have forwarded to you by this conveyance Capt Savage and Inclosed is Invoyce and Bill of loading of the same which I wish well and safe to your hands and to your content. I am forced to advice you of a misfortune attended your small adventure on your owne account vizt the Box with the Sperma Coeti and Castorum was lost the Capt Dying att Sea tis supposed that some of the Saylers supposeing it to bee of value stole it however it was never heard of but the Gourd of Aloes I have received safe and will make the most I can of it. I have entred my protest against the owners of the Ship by vertue of Bill of Loading and have given in to them the value which I could have made of it here and hope I shall have satisfaction for it but am afraid not fully for I am informed in such cases of disasters they allow but two thirds of the value. However I will doe what ever I can and give you credit for the produce and give you an account thereof by the next opertunity. I have sent the shooes for yourself and Pastor; I hade them made on purpose soe hope they will answear your expectations. As to what you write about adventureing in Hatts Haberdashery etc I cannott see it can bee worth while if I hade an Inclination to it to send them att such advance for those kind of goods I am informed by those that deale in them allways sell for 130, 40 or 150 perCent advance or else it never bee worth their while to send them for there is more losse very often upon returnes then that advance. I dont know but by next opertunity I may send you a few Hatts, haveing a Freind that has a parcell to dispose off. If I can agree for them and if soe I will then putt up the 6 payr of Stockins with them. The Case would not hold all the potts but have sent all the species glasses;[1] have sent a smaller Quantity of Myrrh and Jallop by reason of the Extravagant price of them. I have herewith sent back your 2 setts of Dills for the 6£ 4s haveing done all I can to noe purpose to gett the money: and am glad you did not pay for them soe that the losse will not fall upon you. I beleive if you looke over your order you will find you orderd Spanish Dry Liquorish etc what I have now sent is very fine and large and very Carefully packt in earth, tis like to bee very dear this year is likely may come to 12d a pound. The Stoughtons Elixir is the true sort. This is the needfull but hearty Service etc.

[*in margins:* Note to inquire after his Kinsman and send him word.[2] I have inquired after found out and spoken with the Gentleman att the Ship and Ancher in Canon street that your freind desyred me to inquire after and hee is alive and well and told me hee hade very lately writ to his Brother.]

By Capt Savage att the same time writ to Mr Jackson, Mr Nicolls, Mr Greaves and Mr Rand.

1 Species glasses were used to hold the separate ingredients, called 'species,' used in compounding medicines (OED, s.v. 'species').
2 See below, letter 103.

93 MR HABIJAH SAVAGE

London Feb: 18 1715/16

SIR

This serves to inclose Invoyce and bill of loading of your last order which as I advised you before comes in your Brother Capt Savage Ship which I wish well and safe to your hands and every way to your satisfaction. I have charged the Ground Brazzill[1] in this Invoyce which was sent before (and as you very honestly hinted not charged).[2] Everything accept Myrrh and Jallap are agreeable to your Invoyce but they are soe extravagantly Dear there is noe getting of any, Myrrh is worth 12s a pound and if you would give that cannot gett any Quantity. As to the Lockyers pills these sent are the true sort but those you mention that came att 12d a box I am sure are not. I have done all possible for any man to doe to gett them Cheaper and have shewd your letter to the Proprietors and they tooke time to consult togather and att last did consent to take 18d a Box and I am possitive if any one sends them for lesse they must not bee the true sort. I have not bean favoured with any letter from you since that came with the Loggwood in the Whistler Friggatt. I am sorry that I must aquaint you that I cannott gett off your Ambergreace att any price; I have offered it att 12s an ounce and truck for goods for it but no body will meddle with it. If it bee possible I will gett it off but if I cant you can't expect the losse to bee mine for it is not the true thing I thinke veryly and it losses pretty much its smell which was pretty well att first. I am advised by Mr Thomas Greaves that [*in margin:* hee has paid you 24£ on my account. I hope you will take all possible care in the next returnes for really I hade a miserable bargaine in the Loggwood which I have still by me. This is the needfull but etc.]

94 MR THOMAS GREAVES

London Aprill 30 1716

SIR

Your's of November 22 1715 I have receiv'd with Inclosed Invoyce with which I have readily complyed and forwarded to you by this conveyance Capt Osburne which I heartyly wish Safe to your hands and every way to

---

1 Salmon discusses two kinds of brazil: brazilwood used to make red ink, as a tincture good for the face, and as a colouring added to make juleps more appetizing; and a brazil-shrub which he regarded as a medicinal herb which was cold, dry, and astringent (*Pharmacopoeia* 21, 34).
2 Closing parenthesis added

your intire Content and Satisfaction which I have endeavored all I can by putting up the best and Charging the Lowest price of everything that I may incourage a farther and greater Correspondance which I shall readily Embrace. The few Liquids are putt up in the Sand with the Liquorish, the case being to Large have filled it up with Empty viols and Gallypotts which I doubt not will bee useful to you. I have been exact in your order except in the Jallop and wormseeds[1] and Myrrh which are extreamly deare and Scarce and not good neither soe Have onely sent a pound of each instead of 2 pounds and Cochineal[2] of which I have sent none it being near 50s per pound all the rest are exactly according to your direction. I have a Freind in London that will come to Boston in 6 weekes time or thereabouts if any Supply comes in by that time may possibly make up your order by that quantity; I am forced to doe the same by other customers some that have writ for 6 times as much of those things have been forced to send butt a pound of a sort. I understand by your's you have paid Mr Savage the Ballance of the Last account for which I thanke butt have not yet received any advice from him about it. For the future if you can meet with a Bill of exchange or Silver you may transmitt it in that which will save a great deal of trouble. Have sent you the Marble Morter and Glasse morter and pestles and remaine with   Humble Service

95 MR WILLIAM RAND

London Ap[r]ill 30 1716

SIR

Yours of 15 Sept 1715 I am favoured with by Capt Holberton's ship with the Silver sent therein for which I give you thankes and have readily complyed with your order and Invoyce by the same and this serves to Inclose Invoyce and Bill of Loading for the Same sent in Capt Osburne which I heartily wish well and safe to your hands and to your intire content and Satisfaction which I have to the uttmost endeavoured by sending the best of every thing and Chargeing the Lowest price. I was allsoe glad by the same conveyance to hear you had found out the lost things about which I was very much concerned and was allways confident I sent them but you writeing soe possitively could

---

1 Seeds of Turkish wormwood, *Artemisia maritima*, called wormseeds or santonicum, according to Salmon, 'strengthens the Stomach and is vulgarly used to kill and expel Worms' (*Pharmacopoeia* 127). Also see *Ency. Brit.* 24: 195 and Grieve *Modern Herbal* 2: 857-8.
2 Dried bodies of a Mexican and West Indian insect used to make scarlet dye, and also valued as an antidote to poison and in cordials for smallpox, measles, and childhood fevers (Quincy *Complete English Dispensatory* 178). Salmon seems to have confused it with the common ladybird (*Pharmacopoeia* 232).

not tell what to make of it. I have complyed with your order in every thing butt the Myrrh, Sem Santonice,[1] Nardus Indicus[2] (allsoe the Ventrium Scincorum[3] are not sent suppose you Mistook the quantity; they are not to bee gott att present if they were are not sold by the pound bytt by number they are 9 or 10s per dozen and a dozen do not weigh above 3 ounces) which are all extream Scarc and dear soe have sent butt half the quantity and the Synopsis medicina[4] being out of print is nott to bee gott nor the Blagraves Eye water[5] of which I can gett noe account. I have a freind will come to Boston in about 6 week[s] by whom may send what is wanting in this if they are to bee had. The few Liquids that are, are put up in a case by themselves soe that there can bee no mistake. As to returns choose to have it in Silver or in Bills of exchange which you can easyer procure; shall bee gladd to settle a constant annuall correspondance with you from whom you may allways expect and shall receive all imaginable Incouragement (you will find 2 pound of Mirobolans[6] putt up in your case which was done through Mistake; I therefore request you will deliver them to Mr John Nicholls of Boston) from him who is with hearty Service.

96 MR HABIJAH SAVAGE

London Aprill 30 1716

SIR

Yours of January 14 Last per Captain Blair I am favoured with your farther Invoyce which I have forwarded to you by this Conveyance Capt Osburne

---

1 *Sem santonica*, wormseed; see above, letter 94, note 1.
2 *Nardus indicus*, spikenard; see above, letter 1, note 4.
3 *Ventrium scincorum:* bellies of skink. The flesh of a small North African lizard, *Scincus officinalis*, was regarded as an antidote to poison and as an aphrodisiac. It was also considered valuable in a variety of compounds to fight cataracts, epilepsy, and skin ailments, and was used in cosmetics (Quincy *Complete English Dispensatory* 179; Salmon *Pharmacopoeia* 194; *Ency. Brit.* 16: 826).
4 William Salmon's *Synopsis medicinae* (London 1671, 1679-81) is a 1,207-page guide to healing 'astrologically, Galenically and Chymically.' Basically organized according to symptoms, it includes a section on drugs, a list of current drug prices, a discussion of anatomy, and a full index.
5 Probably connected with Joseph Blagrave (1610-82), writer of astrological medicine in the tradition of Culpeper. In addition to his *Supplement or Enlargement to Mr Nich. Culpepper's English Physitian* (London 1674), his medical works include *Blagrave's Astrological Practice of Physick* (London 1671) (DNB).
6 Salmon's *Pharmacopoeia* 122 lists five types of Myrobanus, astringent plum-like fruits of species of *Terminalia*. All were valued as purgatives, two for phlegm, two for choler, and one for melancholy.

and inclos'd a Bill of Loading and Invoyce of the same which I wish well and safe to your hands and every way to your Satisfaction. I allsoe observe what you write about your relinquishing your bargain in the Loggwood upon my advice; how bad a Comodity it was. I am well pleased you did soe for I am sure whoever bought it and Sent it hither his freind would give him Little thankes for it for 'tis not worth 11£ 10s per Tun att most. There is a Neighbour of mine received as much Loggwood this spring from one of your place as cost 400£ there and he declares he did not make cleare of all Charges here above 50£ of it; tho there might bee something extraordinary in that case yet to bee sure it is a very bad comodity. I have mine you sent me by me still And soe am Like to have for any prospect there is of 'tis rice. As to return's I don't see how it is possible to direct, for what is a good comodity att one time in 3 or 4 months is worth nothing allmost and therefore I cannott advice anything better then Bills of Exchange or Silver. I must in a great Measure leave it to your prudent managemennt. Turpentine now beares a good price but perhaps in 3 or 4 months if there comes in a Large quantity it may come to nothing allmost. I hope as you hint you will not refraine giving orders for what you want for the reasons mention'd in you[r] Letter, for tho you may bee sure I shall bee glad of returnes att any time yet had rather the effect should Lye Longer in your hands (where I am satisfied 'tis Safe) then come home att such prodigious losse as everything done. I hope you will have noe ground of complaint of any thing now sent; I thinke all the Volatile spirits are as pungent as possible and everything in there Kind the Best. As to the smalt you not writing whether the Last sent you was what you Liked I have sent you 50 lbs of that Sort and 25 lbs of the Best sort att 2s per lb which am assured is as cheap as the other considering its goodness. Have allsoe sent 2 sorts of manna[1] desire your advice which sort you Like Best and would have of for the future. I desire you will caution the persons that take the goods out of the Ship to bee careful. In the Great case, which is very Large and heavy allsoe, when you open it observe that the spanish Liquorish Lyes Loose att top of the case which pray take of[f] very carefully till you come to the partition of Brown paper next under which Lyes the Gentian putt up Loose; I caution thus that you may not mix them togather. I hope every thing is soe carefully packt that noe damage can come. You will find in each case a Catalogue of the perticulars contain'd therein. This is needful but tenders of hearty Service.

1 Salmon thought manna fell from heaven, regretting that most of it fell in the Orient (*Pharmacopoeia* 147). His view of its use, as a children's laxative and sweet-tasting mask for other medicines, was echoed by later authorities, including Quincy, who knew it was the dried sugary sap of *Fraxinus ornus*, a Mediterranean flowering ash (Quincy *Complete English Dispensatory* 192; *Ency. Brit.* 17: 587-8; Grieve *Modern Herbal* 1:68; Bauer *Potions, Remedies* 16).

97 MR JOHN NICOLLS

London Aprill 30 1716 –

SIR

Yours of Nov. 22 Last I have receiv'd Safe togather with the inclosed Invoyce which I have complyed with and forward'd to you by this conveyance Capt Osburne and this serves to Inclose Invoyce and bill of Loading for the same which wish well to your hands and to your Satisfaction which have endeavoured by putting up the Best of every thing and chargeing them as Low as possible. I received the Silver by your freind Mr Willson as allsoe the pitch but he will bee able att his return to inform you what a Markett it came to. I desire for the future you will if possible make return's in Bills of Exchange or Silver for every thing you have sent yet has come to such a wretched markett as is Enough to discourage farther dealings butt still hope the next will bee Better which makes me willing to proceed. Have sent you the pump with the Glasses[1] and in the Box you will see directions for the use of them printed. Allsoe in the box is putt up the orientall Bezoar which take care you doe not overlooke as allsoe the oyl of cinnamon. What few Liquids there are are putt among the sand with the Liquorish, therefore pray take care you doe nott overlooke them. I shall if I Live write to you again by Mr Willson who will Shortly sail for Boston. I have observed your orders in everything onely the saffron is not extraordinary but then the price charged is not much above one third part of new which is very Scarce and dear. Allsoe wormseeds and Jallop are not to bee had upon any account and cochineal, therefore have sent butt very Little of the former and none of the Latter but if any come in before Mr Willson sails may perhaps send it by him. Allsoe the 2 lbs of Mirobolans which are charged to you were through [*mistake?*][2] packt up with Mr Rands goods whom I have advised of it and desired him to deliver to you which I doubt nott he will. I filled up the empty space in your case with white poppy head[3] which I hope will afford you seeds enough. This is the [*in margin:* needfull but hearty Service.]

1 See above, letter 85, note 10.
2 See above, letter 95.
3 *Papaver somniferum*, the opium poppy, was valued against chest ailments, fluxes, and consumption, as well as for its pain relieving quality, 'and laid to the Head or Feet' was thought to induce sleep (Salmon *Pharmacopoeia* 111, 134).

98 MR WILLIAM ARBUCKLE[1]

London Aug: 16 1716

SIR

Yours of Aprill 16 last past am favoured with and Note the contents thereof allsoe your Invoyce under Covert of your Brother I have received and have forwarded to you by this conveyance Capt Hilliard in the Browne Gally which wish well to your hand and to your content. I shall willingly deale with you on the termes you mention viz 10 Months Credit hope you will not exceed that. I have not yet received your money for the last account but your Brother promises it shall not bee long before I doe. I shall allways carefully observe your orders; all the variations from your present orders were 2 lbs of Jallop instead of 6 lbs because it is not to bee had. I wonder you cannott meet with it where you are for wee have none but what comes from thence.[2] There was lately a parcell of about 400 pound weight entred from your Island but the person demands 14s a pound for the whole parcell. I have serverall orders by mee now for large quantitys of it and send a pound where the order is for 12 lbs. Allsoe Cantharides are growne extreame deare and therefore have sent but a pound instead of 2 lbs. Allsoe the Marble Morters I could not gett but hope to send them the next time your Brother sends any goods which hee talkes will not bee long. The cases not being quite full have putt in some violl Corkes and Empty violls to fill it up. I discoursed Mr Clutterbuck about his Chargeing the Glasse ware to him but hee was not willing to it and it might have occassioned some mistake and therefore have charged them myself and price they cost. [*in margin* I cannott tell what you mean by 2 dozen ornamentall pott with Golded Lybells unlesse you mean Shop potts. Must desyre you to bee more perticuler in your next for I have not sent them now.] I observe what you write about the Mercurialls;[3] I assure you I give the price to a farthing I charge you for them but I have them att our hall[4] where I can depend on the goodnesse of them, I can buy them cheaper of the Towne Chymist but then they are not to be depended on. You shall allways find very

---

1 He went out to Jamaica the previous year. See above, letter 86.
2 Patrick Browne, in *The Civil and Natural History of Jamaica* (London 1756) 166 7, confirms that it was common in Jamaica.
3 Mercurials, mercury compounds, most of which were used to treat syphilis (Salmon *Pharmacopoeia* 265-84, 616).
4 Apothecaries' Hall, Water Lane, London, meeting place and dispensatory of the Society of Apothecaries of London

Canded usage from me in all respects and if you will bee content with the other sort shall have them somewhat Cheaper. I desyre allways you will bee as perticuler as you can in your orders which shall bee punctually observed. I was greatly surprized to find you mention not one word of the Affayr about Perkins[5] nor have I heard one word from either of those 2 Gentlemen I sent the power of Attourney to; mythinkes tis strange if they would not engage in it that they would not favour me with a letter whether they would or not. I intreat the favour of a letter by the next ship about it and if you can informe yourself what circumstances Perkins is in and whether Dr Tredway have payd the 200£ to Perkins. For if theyr Gentlemen will not engage in it must intreat yourself or some other person [*in margin*: you shall think fitt to advice me to to send over another power of Attourny to for I cannott loose soe much money without great damage. I begg your answeare to this by the first Shipping And pray if Mrs Stiles bee liveing give my hearty Service to her and accept the same yourself from Sir   Yours etc.

99 MESSIEURS CRAWFORD & POYNTZ

London Aug 18 1716

GENTLEMEN

With the advice of Mr Waterhouse Fernly I wrote to you Aug 25 last and therewith sent you a power of Attourney to sue for a Debt of 200 Sterling due to me from Mr Thomas Perkins since which I have never been favoured with one line in answeare to it which mythinks is very strange. If you hade not pleased to have engaged in it it would have been noe great trouble to have advised me you would not. I should not have troubled you if Mr Fernly hade not advised me to it and assured me you would undertake it and I did not expect you should doe it without a reward. Tis much a whole yeare, within a few days, should now passe and not one step that I know of taken in it, to bee sure if the Debt were precarious then tis soe if not worse now. What I therefore now desyre of you is if you will not engage in it that you will by the first shipping advice me of it and returne the power of Attourny that I may employ some other person. This I hope you will not deny me and you'l oblige etc.   Yours

5 See above, letter 86.

100 MR HABIJAH SAVAGE

London Aug: 25 1716

SIR

Yours of May 9th last per Capt English am favoured with, with Invoyce of
Bill of loading for 46 barrills of Traine oyle which have received safe and for
which returne you hearty thankes. It come to a tollerable markett and I believe was as good a Comodity as you could have sent. I sold it for about 96£
sterling, but there was allmost 3 Barrells leakt out and near 20£ Charges
upon it which brings it to about 76£. I dont know anything else could have
done better and if you thinke well should like to have more of it if not to
deare. I have by this Conveyance sent you 2 lbs Jallop and 3 lbs Sem Santonici; they are putt up in a Case of Mr Bartons. I have writt to him to deliver
them to you on demand. They are both soe extravagant Scarce and Dear
there is none to bee gott att any price. There was lately a small parcell
brought in and the person that imported it askes 14s a pound for the whole
parcell, and wormeseed there are none to bee bought otherwise I should have
sent your whole quantity. I give you this advice that you may put your price
upon them accordingly. Allsoe would advice you that Senna[1] is risen very
much, the Parliament have layd a new duty of above 1s a pound upon it and
wee are obliged to pay for what stock wee have by us,[2] soe that you must
never expect to have it come for lesse then 3s if for soe little. I am glad you
hade soe good a stock that you will not want againe quickly. This the needfull
but humble Service from Sir,   Yours   JC

101 MR WILLIAM RAND

Aug 25 1716

SIR

This onely serves to aquaint you that I have by this conveyance etc. They are
what your former Invoyce ordered but were left behind then; they are put up
in A Case with Mr Thomas Bartons goods who will deliver them to you upon

---

1 Dried leaflets of North African species of cassia constituted senna, a common purgative given as
a powder or infused in Rhine wine. Because it caused griping, it was not taken alone (Salmon
Pharmacopoeia 91).

2 By 1 Geo. 1 c. 43 an earlier exemption for senna was stopped. Stocks on hand exceeding 20 lbs.
were to be taxed (*Statutes* 13: 286).

demand. The Blagraves Eye water and Salmons Synopsis are not to bee gott And the Nardus Indicus is att an extravagant price; tis worth above 40s a pound and not good neither soe have not sent but hope you may meet with it there. I am inclined to Believe Mr Barton can help you to some for I once sent him a parcell which I believe hee has not yet used. This is the needful but etc from Sir   Yours etc.

102 MR THOMAS GREAVES

London Aug 25 1716

This onely serves to you that I have sent you (Rad Julapis,[1] Myrrhe, Sem Santon[2] an 1lb, Coccinella[3] 4 ozs) by this conveyance. They come in a case of Mr Thomas Barton who will deliver them to you on demand. I have writt to him to doe soe they are what was left behind of your former order; they are very deare all of them but can noe way help it they are not to bee gott for any price now. I hope you have received your former parcell of Aprill 30 safe and to your content. As to returnes if you can't gett a Bill for the sume if you please you may doe as you did before, pay it to Mr Savage, tho if you can meet with a Bill hade rather then give him the trouble. This is the needfull from Sir   Yours   JC

103 MR THOMAS BARTON

London Aug 25: 1716

SIR

Yours of June 16 last I am favoured with with another Invoyce which I have put up and now forward to you by Capt Moses Thomas which I wish safe to your hands and to your Content. I observe the Contents; I could make noe other termes than I advised you of before with the owners of Capt Holbertons Ship tho I did as much as if the affayr were my owne. I have sent you 2 payr of Shoes made according to your order and hope they will fitt well. As to what you write of my not observeing your orders and sending you Species glasse for Gallypotts,[1] I have to this letter pin'd a Line of your letter wherein

1 Jalap root
2 *Sem santonica*, wormseed
3 Cochineal

1 This presumably means that the glass containers for unmixed ingredients were received rather than the glazed earthenware gallypots used for keeping mixed medicines.

you will see whether you or I were mistaken and for the Liquorish I beleive if it bee uselesse to you Mr Savage will take it off you for hee always sends for Spanish Liquorish; I have sent him severall times large quantitys of it. Gum Senica[2] being now very cheap I have doubled your order and sent 56 instead of 28 lbs within this 2 yeare it [*dropped?*] 6£ 5s a hundred. Allso have added to your Invoyce 20 lbs Suc Glycyrrhiz Hyspan,[3] it is extraordinary fine and the Cheapest I ever bought in my life. I bought a large Quantity of it, don't doubt but it will bee acceptable to you; but Jallop is intollerable dear soe have sent lesse of it, the Merchants that import it ask 14s a pound for it. Wee are att a sad passe for Druggs most of them bee very scarce and Senna which was the onely thing allmost that was cheap is now growne Dear by reason of a tax layd by the Parliament upon it of above 12d a pound. I have sent but 6 lbs of the Distilled verdigreece[4] by reason I feare you are not apraised of the value of it, in some places they askt 16s a pound in others 14s. I bought att the cheapest place I could meet with; it is they informe me a very chargeable and dangerous thing to make. I suppose that quantity will serve you till you can have more which if you desyre you may have what you please. The Case being to large have filled it up with 3 grosse of vialls sorted which I hope will bee usefull to you. And now I must begg your excuse for troubling soe farr which I did not well know how to prevent. You will find in opening the case 4 small paper parcells, directed to Mr Savage, Mr Nicolls, Mr Rand, and Mr Greaves, which I intreat the favour of you to deliver to them each on demand and let them pay each what you thinke is reasonable toward the Freight. They were small matters that were not to bee hade when I sent there maine parcells, and was afraid if sent alone they would bee lost. I hope you'l excuse this trouble. I have found out your Kinsman the Musicall Instrument Maker who is well and seemingly in a Flourishing Condition; hee lives at the Crowne in Thredneedle street near the Exchange. If I can I will gett a letter from him to you. Sir you will find these goods charged but att 65[5] perCent advance, for Mr Savage and some others have brought me downe to that standard and I cant satisfye myself to let you pay dearer then other people with whom I have dealt soe many yeares. I hope every thing will please you haveing taken all the care about them that possibly I could. This is the needfull but hearty service etc.

2 Gum senica is the gum of a variety of acacia native to Senegal (OED).
3 *Suc glycyrrhiz hyspan* is syrup of Spanish licorice. See above, letter 9, note 2.
4 Verdigrease, substance obtained by applying acetic acid to copper. It was valued for cleansing open sores, particularly sores in children's mouths (Quincy *Complete English Dispensatory* 260, 227; OED).
5 Changed in MS from 75

104 MR HABIJAH SAVAGE

London Sept: 28 1716

SIR

Above is Copy of what I sent you by poor Capt Thomas who in a violent storme while in the Downes was drove from his Anchor and cast away and every person in his Ship drowned but one and the Ship staved all to peices and her Cargoe lost; She hade about 20 passengers in her. You will heare enough of that sad providence. Since the above I have been favoured with yours of July 7 per Capt Loyd with advice you hade shipt 20 Barrills of Turpentine in Capt Playsted who is not yet heard of allsoe your small Invoyce which have forwarded to you by this Conveyance Capt Eve which wish better Successe then the former mett with. I hope for the future you will bee willing to allow the Ensurance which for the future I shall allways make for it being low in time of peace I thinke tis better then run such risques. I have Ensured those things now sent tho theyr beeing but a Trifle have not charged it to your account. I am informed by others that trade to your Country that they never run any risque outward and I thinke tis but highly reasonable for what dealings I have in England I run noe hazzard or losse after they are delivered to the Carryer; if they should bee stole or any way lost or damaged it lyes upon the person that sent for them. I observe what you note of the Suc Kermes[1] I hope you will find it, I am sure it was put up. And for the Spanish saffron I writ you word it was ordinary and therefore the price was according and sure it must bee worth what I charged for it. I am afraid by what I can understand yet that if the Turpentine dos arrive safe it will come to a very poor markett. This is the needful but etc.

105 MR THOMAS GREAVES

London Sept 28 1716

SIR

Above is Coppy of what I writt you by poor Capt Thomas who in a Storme [*blot:* etc?], since which I am favoured with yours of June 27 with another In-

---

1 *Sucus kermes*, syrup of kermes. Kermes is a species of scale insect, *Coccidae*, which was a source of crimson dye until the introduction of cochineal for that purpose. Until 1714 the animal nature of kermes was unknown, and both Salmon *Pharmacopoeia* 60 and 162 and Robert James *Medicinal Dictionary* in the 1740s still talk of them as berries of the Mediterranean oaks which the kermes inhabited. Medicinally they were valued as cordial, sudorific, astringent, and antidote to poison. See also *Ency. Brit.* 15: 756-7.

voyce which I have Shipt you in Capt Eve Invoyce and bill of Loading of which comes inclosed which wish better successe then the former. Indeed it was well I hade not your order sooner for if I hade I hade sent them in Capt Thomas in whom I have severall parcells etc. You observe I have charged Ensurance which designe to doe for the future to all I deal with etc. If you can make returns in oyl I should like it well if not please to make it any otherwise as you can most conveniently. This is the needfull but etc.

106 MR WILLIAM RAND

Sept: 28 1716 –

SIR

I wrote largely to you Aug 25 last and then sent you Sem Santonici 2 lb, Myrrh 1 lb, Stinces[1] 2 dozen, Coccinelle 4 ozs in all to the value of 3£-15-1 in poor Capt Thomas who etc. His losse was but a few days agoe soe could not possible procure the same things againe for I was greatly troubled to get the Stinces before. I am greatly concerned for the disapoyntment on your account as well as my owne and designe what I send abroad for the future to ensure etc. This is the last ship that will sayle this season soe that you must not expect to heare againe before the Spring and by that time I hope shall heare from you againe. Which is the need full att present but hearty Service etc.

107 MR THOMAS BARTON

Sept: 28 1716 –

SIR

Above is Copy of what I writt you with Invoyce and bill of Loading in Poor Capt Thomas who etc. I thinke you cant in reason expect the losse should all fall upon me when I hade shipt them by your order and I am very well assured that is the termes all other people trade upon to run no risque outward. And for the time to come I resolve to Ensure all I send out which in times of peace is not above 2 and ½ perCent which I thinke you nor noe other person can thinke much to allow. Mr Leigh told me since this losse hapned hee never runs any risque out that hee hade severall hundred pounds in that Ship but hade ensured it all and Charged it to his Customers that he has not a penny damage. Therefore since this sad providence has hapned I thinke it

---

1 Obsolete form of skink (OED). See above, letter 95, note 3.

but reasonable that both partys should beare their proportion; the prime cost without the Advance You see by the Invoyce is 33-18-11½ which I hope you will bee willing to allow one half of and I will beare the other and soe shall charge your account with but 16-19-6. This losse hapning but a few days agoe it was impossible to provide the same things againe to send by this ship which is the last that will sayle this season, soe that you must not expect them before the spring but by the first that sayles in the Spring I shall not fayle (God willing)[1] to send them againe. I am now favoured with yours of July 21 by Capt Thwaites with 300 ozs Silver which I have received safe and thanke you for it. Hee was allsoe in that storme and escaped very narrowly, being lost heard nothing of him for 6 days after which you must Imagine made me very unEasye; I hade allsoe concernes in Severall other Shipps that were in danger but thanke God hade noe other Losse but in Capt Thomas. This is the needfull etc.

108 MR WILLIAM PHILLIPS[1] BARBADOS

London Nov: 8 1716

SIR

Yours of July 26 last I am favoured with with inclosed Invoyce for a parcell of Druggs and Medicines which I have taken the first occasion to putt up and now forward to you by this Conveyance Capt Gould, which I wish safe to your hand and every way to your Content. Inclosed conteines Invoyce and bill of loading of the same. You will find every thing sent but the Mace which cannot bee gott; I tryed att many places but none hade any. Att one place onely I could have gott 2 ounces but must have given 5s for the 2 ounces. I hope the disapoyntment in the want of that cannott bee much. Everything else is very good and charged as low as possible tho some Druggs are very Dear as Jallop and Cantharides and Severall others but you shall allways find all the Freindly and Candid usage you can desyre and shall bee very glad this may bee the beginning of a settled yearly Correspondance. Just now lookeing over your letter I find one thing omitted vizt the sweet powder[2] which was not in your Invoyce, I am sorry for it but indeed [did] not see it.

1 Closing parenthesis added

1 Son of Dr William Phillips
2 Sweet powder was perfumed powder used as cosmetic (OED). A recipe for sweet powder from dried roses, from 1682, is quoted in E.S. Rohde *The Old English Herbals* (London 1922) 180.

Hope if I live to send againe shall not omitt it. I have you see charged the Advance but att 45 perCent which as you write I did last yeare to Dr Lucas but I assure you that was the lowest and the first time I ever sent any goods att soe low advance and I am sure the returnes Mr Adams sent I shall loose greatly by, for the Sugars hee sent are very ordinary and very low, have not yet sold them nor know not when I shall. You may depend if I can find the least incouragement shall bee willing to correspond with you. One thing you'l observe which perhaps youle wonder a little att. I have charged Insurance which I think is highly reasonable and indeed have resolved to doe soe to all I deale with and have done soe to my Chapmen in New England. You know what a severe losse I hade in Capt Lassells and Another att the same time and this yeare have hade a very great losse in a Ship cast away in a storme. Now in time of peace the Ensurance is small and therefore resolve for the future to Ensure all and I hope this will satisfye you of the reasonablenesse of my soe doing. I desyre in your returnes if it bee in Sugar it may bee very good tho you give some what dearer, for ordinary Sugar pay the same Freight, Customes, etc. as the worst and the ordinary is much harder to dispose of; a good Comodity will goe off att any time. Would bee glad if one hoggshead were white Sugars for that would serve me for my owne use; or if you could meet with any Aloes would bee glad of some. I leave it to you to act for my interest as you can. I was greatly concerned to heare of the death of your father, but am glad to find hee has a son soe capable to succeed him in his busynesse and heartyly wish you successe and prosperity in that and all other of your concernes. [in margin: This is the needfull but hearty Service etc.]

109 MR GEORGE STEWART

London Feb 2 [blurred: 26?] 1716 [/17]

SIR

Yours of Aug. 1 1716 I am favoured with, with a Small Invoyce which I have put up and forwarded to you by this Conveyance Capt Beard. Inclosed is Invoyce and Bill of Loading of the same which wish well and safe to your hands and to your full satisfaction. Every thing is sent in the proportion you ordered accept the Sem Santonici of which you ordered 10 lbs and have sent but 3 lbs by reason of the extreame Scarcenesse and dearnesse of it and not very fresh neither. I hope that may supply your present occasions till more come. I observe what you write about your orders to Capt Thwaites to receive some moneys due to you att Edinborough and have severall times spoke with him about it, and he tells mee hee forwarded your letters thither but never received any answeare back whether they would pay it or not soe see but little reason to expect any thing from them nor have I heard any thing of any goods from you which your letter mentions you designed to send me and speake as if you hade actually bought them. I cannott well tell how to reconcile this matters: but however being unwilling to disapoynt you have sent your goods and therefore hope and expect, if you have not sent any effects before this arrives, that you will take the first opertunity of remitting effects to Ballance the former and this account. I intreat you will not disapoynt me etc. and shall allways take perticuler care to oblige you in every order receive from you who am etc.   JC

110 MR JOHN NICOLLS OF BOSTON

Mar: 1 1716/17

SIR

Yours of November 22 last I am favoured with, [*with*] your inclosed Invoyce which I have put up and forwarded to you by this conveyance Capt Beard, Invoyce and Bill of Loading of which comes inclosed which wish well to your hand and to your full Content which I heartyly wish. Your proportions are observed in every thing I thinke but the Jallop and Wormeseed of which have sent a lesse quantity by reason of the extreame dearnesse of them but hope in some time they will bee somewhat Cheaper. Hope this may Serve your present occasions. I have sent every thing good and charged very low onely the Senna is dearer then the last by reason of a very great new duty layd on it, which will allways keepe it as dear if not dearer. I received the Castor by Capt Osbourne and have given you Credit for it; it was vastly dryed in and lost in weight but as the custome was saved it did as well as any thing you could send; allsoe received the money by the same conveyance. I have allsoe received your kind Token of Cranberrys very safe and good for which self and spouse returne our hearty thankes. As to what you write of the oyle of Pennyroyall I feare I shall never dispose of it and soe I told Mr Willson when hee left; tis not used much, and a great deal of it comes off in distilling the herb. I have neare 2 Quarts by me that I have saved. If I can meet with any one will buy it will doe the best I can to doe it. Hope you'l make returnes with as much speed as you can, if you could meet with oyle I beleive it would doe as well as any thing. Tho everything is very bade, I hope you'l doe the best you can etc. and you'le oblige etc.   Yours   JC

writt to him about the Ensurances.

111 MR THOMAS BARTON ATT SALEM

Mar: 2: 1716/17

SIR

This serves to inclose Invoyce and Bill of Loading for your Invoyce last yeare repeated againe, and the small addition to it by your order in yours of Dec. 29 per Capt Chadder which I wish better Successe then the former and hope will prove to your satisfaction. I hade put up the Distilled Verdigreace before your letter arrived being just ready to Ship the goods but unpackt them againe upon the receipt thereof and have now omitted it. Hope this Ship will sayle in a few days soe chose to take the first opertunity but in 14 days Capt Lithered will sayle by whom shall write againe more att large and answear all your Long complaineing lettter. In the meantime Subscribe myself Yours etc.

[12 March 1716/17]

I am now come to March 12 and take this opertunity by Capt Lythered to inclose second Bill of loading and Invoyce of those things sent in Capt Beard and according to promise there to consider the contents of your long letter of Dec. 29 last wherein you first wonder I should ask you to beare any part in the losse in Capt Thomas which, after all you write, I must owne I can not see but is very reasonable and your saying you give such advance seemes to me no answear att all because the advance you give dos not answeare to the losse on goods by returnes if they goe and come safe, nor nothing neare the advance that other goods sell att which I know many of them sell att 200 perCent and upwards. You desyre me to let you into the mystery. I assure I know none in favour of myself but beleive upon the strictest search I can possibly make into all the trade that ever I hade to New England in all my life I never cleared 6 perCent for my money which I am sure is not worth while haveing soe much fateique and trouble about it. And really think scarce any but myself (who hade all ways a great inclination to trafick abroad which I have a long time done but really B[eleive] I had better let alone) would venture any more after soe many losses both by the Hazards of the Sea and upon returne of goods. I am sure I know many of my owne trade who never traded for a quarter of what I have done nor imployed a quarter of the stock that I have that yet have gott 4 times what I am worth. I thinke the matter is plaine even to demonstration that if a man sells his goods att 65 perCent advan[ce] and looses 80 perCent by returnes, as I am sure for the most part I doe, must bee a great looser especially when 4 parts in 5 of these goods are Druggs or other things bought with ready money. Indeed for Compounds it may doe pretty well but you know they are farr the least part of your orders. As for all Drugs and things out of my owne way I am sure I have taken more paines then any one in London besides would have done to Apply the Makers or Importers that soe I might buy everything att the best hand and all with ready money such as the oyle Cloth, Gallypotts etc. and all the Colours. If you hade been here yourself with ready money you could not have bought them Cheaper nor noe cheape[r?] by 5 perCent as I charge you. And for saying if I did not like to send them on these termes I might have lett it alone tis true I was not under any neccessity of sending them but I was unwilling to disapoynt you not knowing how urgent your occasions might bee for them. As to your saying who askt me to bear a part in the losse of the Sperma Coeti and Castor I thinke there is noe Comparison between 40£ losse and 4 or 5 pound losse which sume I beleive your losse did not amount to for I have received 5£ 2s Sterling for the Sperma Coeti and Castor of the Owners of the Ship and have given you Credit for it which was the uttmost I could gett. And I am sure if you hade been hear yourself you could not have gott more for I tooke more paines about it then if it hade been intyrely my owne. I am confident I never cleared by all your dealing with me soe much as that parcell amounted to. And for the Aloes, I have sold it at 9£ Sterling a hundred and there was 59 [lbs.] nett of it which amounts to 4£ 14s 9d Sterling which I have given you Credit for. I Assure you tho I have not charged you insurance yet I have to all other people I have sent goods to by the same ship and am resolved soe to doe for the future for I am sure the profitts will not beare such losses as must reasonably bee expected if it were onely from the danger of the Sea and not time of warr, which is not like long to bee our case for wee were going into a new warr with Sweden and their Pryvateers are out thick allready in our narrow Seas. I designed noe harme in mentioning Mr L[eigh] and if it gave you offence I beg your pardon; I cannott tell anything of his way of trade more then from his owne Mouth and I was in the house when hee received his money for the goods hee Ensured on Capt Thomas. I am for my part soe indifferent in the matter that if you choose it rather will take 10 perCent in Sterling money paid here free of all hazzard and Advance nothing att all on them and I believe I should be more a gainer by that then by Anything I have done yet. And I dare say 10 perCent is lesse then any tradesman in London will sell his goods for and trust a year or more, in lesse time then which I cant suppose returnes can bee made. And therefore I retort your owne argument back upon you, doe by me as you would bee done by yourself, and I desyre noe more and If I know my owne heart I designe and Endeavour to make that the rule of my practice. What you may buy there I cannott tell. Wee have abundance of people here take up great quantitys of Goods and then breake and run away beyond Sea and never pay for them. Now such people may well sell good pennyworth but if they buy them and pay for them I am well assured no one can or will cheaper then I doe for none of the trade I am sure bys his good[s] better or pay for them better. I shall take care to avoid sending any parcells to you for other people; I did not know it could bee so troublesome. As you say you like your tradeing with me very well And I assure you I doe the same by you and never did and trust I never shall have any occasions to complaine of you. I have lookt over your Account and find I have charged you a great deal lower then other people. I am very glad you did not send the Juice of Liquorish for if you hade the Custome would have been more then tis worth. What wee have here is all run and the Custome saved or else it could never bee sold for the price it is. I am now favoured with yours of Jan 15 by Capt Eve and shall in a few days send you the 4 things you therein order by the hands of a pertickuler Freind[1] that comes over passenge[r] in Capt Chadder who will sayle in 10 or 12 days. This is the needfull but hearty Service etc.

112 MR WILLIAM LITTLE

London Apr: 17 1717

SIR

Yours of January 10 last I have received and observe the Contents thereof. And if you please to consult the Contents of mine to you of March 5, 1710/-11, of Aprill 5, 1712 And of Aug 25, 1712 (of all which letters I keepe Coppys by me) your wonder will cease that I have not sent you the Ballance of your account which I thinke is fully done there. But, however, that you may have noe objections, I have inclosed it againe by which you see I am in your debt but 7d and yet have charged none of the expense I was att about getting 100£ Ensured on Capt Kent according to your desyre about which I was att a considerable charge beside a vast deal of time and paines and tho I did not gett it done (as it was well I did not as it proved that you had noe goods on board the Ship) yet the time and expence was as much and more as if I had done it.

1 Philip Hedman; see below, letter 113.

I doe not remember that I ever received from you any letter since that wherein was the Certificate for the Turpentine. If I hade I thinke I should have answeared it before for I cannott Charge myself with any neglect in that affayr. I confesse there was a very uncomon series of disapoyntment attended that small concernes wee hade togather, but I cannott see any reason why you should reflect on me for that, for I hade goods of my owne on board the same Ship that suffered the same fate. I should have been glad if none of these disasters hade hapned, but as they did I could noe way help it. I shall allways endeavour to deal by you and every one else I have any concernes with as I would bee done bye. I have allsoe herewith sent your Brother Thomas Littles account by the ballance of which hee is due to me 5£ 11s 8½d in Sterling money here which hope his Executors will take care to remitt me. I never advanced anything on any goods I sent him but hee allways paid me in Sterling money here. If there bee any farther [*in margin*: Satisfaction you desyre or I can give you, you may freely demand it. This is the needful etc.

Sent by Capt Chadder]

113 MR GEORGE JACKSON

May 15 1717

SIR

I have waited year after year in expectation you would have performed your repeated promises of paying me the money you have soe many years unjustly deteined from me. I therefore give you this advice that I have given a full proof of my Debt and power of Attourney to Mr Phillip L Hedman Merchant in Boston (who has been some time here and returnes by this Conveyance to settle in Boston) to receive it of you and give you a full discharge. And in case of not complyance, to sue and prosecute you for it. Therefore hope you will prevent any trouble to yourself or him by a ready Complyance and if any trouble comes you must blame yourself and not me for I am sure I have hade patience enough and have waited longer then you or any one else would on me. The sume you know is 56-16-2¼ Sterling not New England money. Your complyance herein will Oblige Sir   Yours   JC

[*in margin*: Att the same time wrote to Mr Savage that I hade shipt his goods on Capt Eve who would Sayle in a few days.]

114 MR THOMAS BARTON

London May 30 1717

SIR

I have writt largely to you by Capt Lithered to which I referr you allso by Capt Beard with allsoe Invoyce and bill of Loading of what good I sent you by him. This cheifly serves to conteine Invoyce and Bill of Loading of a Small Box conteining what you formerly ordered now sent by Capt Mordecai Eve. There is but 3 lbs of the Gum Elemni[1] it being exceeding scarce and deare hade much a doe to get that. You will observe this account is valued New England money 50 perCent being advanced on them and noe more. I wish them well and safe to your hands and hope to heare from you speedyly and receive some effects and farther orders which shall bee complyed with by Sir   Yours etc.

115 MR HABIJAH SAVAGE

London June 3 1717

SIR

Yours of Jan. 18 last past per Capt Pittman I have received with inclosed Catalogue of Medicines which I have put up and as I advised you by Capt Chadder have sent you by this conveyance in the Griffin, Capt Eve which I wish well and safe to your hands and to your Content and satisfaction. There are some few things not sent att all by reason they are not to bee hade att all and of some other a smaller Quantity then you writt for (and account of which have inclosed) by reason of their scarcity etc., which I designe to forward to you within a Month by one of the next ships that sayles. I have sent you 4 lbs of English Saffron onely 2 pounds is not quite soe fine as the other 2 pound but Spanish would have been 32[s.?] a pound and not half soe good. I have taken all the care and paines possible in packing them and everything in its kind is very good and fresh. I doubt you will not receive the Spicknard by the next; there is none to bee gott att any price. I sold it to The Drugsters here in Towne as long as I hade any for 40s a pound but have none left nor

1 Gum Elemi, a white rosin from an Ethiopian tree, dissolves readily in oils and converts easily into an oil. It was valued for healing wounds, especially head wounds, and as a mild and agreeable laxative (Salmon *Pharmacopoeia* 144; OED, s.v. 'elemi').

doe not know where to gett a pound in London. I shall write to you again by next conveyance. Remaine with hearty Service.   Yours etc.   JC

Advised him about the Ensurance and returnes.

116 MR JOHN PHYLLIPS¹ ATT BARBADOS

June 12 1717

SIR

Yours of Aprill 15 last past am favoured with and Inclosed Invoyce and observe the Contents thereof But cannott understand what you meane by Expecting I should send your goods without advance. Tis what I never heard of before nor never reckond soe small advance as I did on your Brothers last year. Sure you can never desyre I should send good without advance and loose 50 perCent by returnes as I am sure I have all along done; I am sure this is the way to sell and live by the losse. And for your accepting againest Ensurance and saying you see noe reason for it, if you will have them on your owne riske you may but I am resolved to run none; have hade a great many severe losses and Ensurance is small now. I remember the last parcell I ever sent your father was not ensured and lost and hee would not allow me a farthing towards it by which I am sure I lost more then ever I gained by all the tradeing I ever hade with him. You seeme to bee quite wrong in your notian about advance. You write your Brother William wonders I should advance on them when they were sent emediately to him and not to Mr Adams. Now all you save by haveing directly consignd to yourself is the Commission and not the advance which I ever charged to every person I ever delt with and for the most part 20 perCent or at least 50 perCent more then I charged your Brother. I thinke tis plaine to demonstration that without advance who ever trades must bee undone when the losse on returnes is soe vastly great; the last parcell of Sugar I received from Mr Adams I lost att least 60 perCent by this. I thinke is sufficient to satisfye you and therefore shall say noe more of it But send this to aquaint you I am inclineable enough to settle a Correspondance with you and designe to putt up and forward to you as soon as possible both yours and your Brother Mr Thomas's Invoyces upon these Conditions vizt all the Medicines and Druggs att the lowest ready money price here without any advance on condition of my running noe risque out nor home but you to pay

1 Son of Dr William Phillips of Barbados (d. 1716) and brother of William and Thomas Phillips, all of whom were correspondents of Cruttenden

for them here in 9 months time from their Shipping in Sterling money either by Bills of Exchange or goods which you please. And for the other goods which are out of my way which I must buy with ready money those to bee paid for here att 12 perCent advance in Sterling money allsoe att 9 months end and I shall take all Imaginable care to buy Everything att the best hand and as good as possible and I am sure 12 perCent is lesse then any tradesman will lay out his money and trust 9 Months and thinke you can have noe objections against that. And upon these Conditions you may expect your orders as soon as possible and please to advice your Brother Thomas of the same. And your Brother William of what I write that if hee has not allready sent effects hee may doe it as soon as possible. If att any time you consigne effects to me I shall dispose of them to the best advantage I can possible and give your Account Credit for it. This I hope will satisfye you.   Remaine etc.
forwarded by Capt Sprigmore

[*in margin*: Note: Writ by the same Ship Large to Mr Adams and pressed him earnestly to Ballance my Account and allso Sister Braggs and send the Effects by the first oppertunity.]

117 TO MR JOHN COMPTON ATT MR JOSEPH THORNES NEAR THE TOWN DOCK IN BOSTON IN NEW ENGLAND

July 31 1717

SIR

Inclosed is a letter from Mr John Taylor to whom you owe some money on an account of some goods he sent by you when here Aprill 10th, 1714 to the value of 35£ which you were to sell by Commission for him. Now I have lent him a large sum of money and among other things have your note left in my hands as a security. Now you see by his letter hee has directed you to make the returnes of the Ballance of the account which you have in your hands to me And emediately upon the receipt thereof I will deliver up your Note to your Cousin Norris or to any other person you shall apoynt here to receive it and give you (in which Mr Taylor allsoe shall joyne) a full discharge of all demands. Thercfore I desyre and hope you will by the very first opertunity make the returnes in such comoditys as you thinke will best answeare. I believe oyle will doe as well as any thing or Silver if not to high in the Exchange. You must remember in the returnes from your Country there is very great losse therefore hope you sold the goods att proportionable advance. I hope you will bee as expeditious as possible I haveing been allready a great while out of my money and have noe consideration for the loan of it. Please to direct for me att the Green Dragon in Newgate Street, London and if you write to him you may inclose it in mine. Your complyance herein will oblige   Yours etc.   JC

118 MR HABIJAH SAVAGE

London July 30 1717

SIR

My last to you of June 3rd last per Capt Eve with Invoyce and Bill of Loading of Parcell of wares shipt you by him hope you have received in good order; have herewith inclosed a second bill of Loading and Invoyce of the same goods. Alsoe according to my promise then, this serves to inclose Invoyce and Bill of Loading of a farther parcell of goods for you being the remainder of the former Invoyce which I hinted to you then I should Shortly forward to you. Every thing is now sent but the 2 lbs of Spicknard which is not to bee gott for any price whatever and the 20 lbs wormseeds of which have sent but 3 lbs they being extreame Scarce and Dear. I know but of one person in London that has any and hee gave 7s a pound the first Cost for the whole parcell that was imported. I beleive you will scarce ever have the Senna soe cheape againe; I did not expect to have gott it myself soe cheape by farr concidering the vast duty it pays but hapned to meet with a parcell reasonable. The Juniper Berrys are not very good but they are the best I have att present; have therefore charged them accordingly. All the other perticulers are very fine and good. In lookeing over your things you will find a little paper (containeing onely 2 lbs Crocus Mettallorum)[1] directed to Mr John Nicholls which I beg the favour you will lett one of your servants deliver to him. I hade nothing else to send him and was afraid it might bee lost alone; hope you'l excuse the trouble which I would not otherwise have given you. Hope this fall to heare farther from you. This is the needful att present but etc.

119 MR THOMAS BARTON

Lond July 31: 1717

SIR

I have allready [written] by Capt Cary that I have received yours of May 24 per Capt Lythered and allsoe according to your order sent you 40 Bookes ie

---

1 Sulphurated oxide of antimony, rarely used medicinally, but part of a tartar emetic, and used to make antimonial wine, according to Edward Kremers *American Pharmaceutical Documents, 1643-1780* (Madison 1944) 23

1000 Leaves of Gold[1] by Capt Cary which hope you will receive safe; sent the Capt receipt for it inclosed in that letter. This serves to inclose Invoyce and Bill of Loading for the rest of your small order now sent by the Swallow, Capt Walkers which wish well to you. I never expected I should have mett with any more Senna soe cheap as this therefore have sent a little more then your order, I cannott thinke but the next will bee Dearer. I am very glad to heare all disputes are like to have an end which I assure you will bee very pleasing to me. This is the needfull but hearty Service, etc.

120 TO MR JOHN PHYLLIPS ATT BARBADOS

Sept: 6: 1717

SIR

In persuance of my Advice and promise to you of June 12 last past per Capt Springmore (which I hope came Safe to your hands) This serves to inclose Invoyce and Bill of Loading of the parcell of goods in your order now sent by Capt Combs in the Grocer Friggott which I wish well and safe to your hand and hope they will every way prove to your intyre content and Satisfaction, which I have as much as possible endeavoured. You will observe according to the conditions I then proposed I have made 2 Invoices: one of the things I have bought with ready money, and the other of Druggs and Medicines. The latter noe advance is made upon but they are charged as low as wee sell them for ready money to any Chapmen here the other being all bought with ready money have advanced 12 perCent upon them which I am sure is lesse by farr then any one else would have done beside. I have taken all possible care in the buying of Everything and showed your directions to Every one that I bought them off and hope they will soe farr please you as to incourage a farther Correspondance. I desyre you to bee carefull when you open the Cases that you doe not overlooke any of the small parcells for I am sure every thing is putt up but onely the 2 Earthen plates which I forgott but have put up in your Brother Thomas Case, and the pil Panchymagogis[1] which I cannott meet with the receipt of anywhere. I hope you'l make returnes by the Spring ships and remember that I run noe risque out or home. This is the need full but hearty Service, etc.   JC

---

1 Gold leaf had medicinal uses, but in this quantity was probably used for dental work. See St Julien R. Childs 'A South Carolina Physician, 1693-1697' *J. Hist. of Med.* 26 (1971): 19.

1 *Panchymagogis*, a universal vegetable purge, valued against scurvy, dropsy, gout, jaundice, etc. (Salmon *Pharmacopoeia* 454). He also refers to an elixir and a pill (609).

121 TO MR WILLIAM PHYLLIPS

Sept: 6 1717

SIR

Yours of June 5th last per Capt Gabriell I am favoured with, with Invoyce and Bill of Loading for one hoggshead of Sugar and one Gourd Aloes which is come safe and, tho I have not yet seen either, for which I give you in hearty thankes. Sugars are very low here; feare it will come to very dull markett but hope what Clayd Sugar will doe better which you promised to send in a Month's time. I have according to your desyre sent you by this Conveyance what farther Medicines you writ for as you see hereby, and because the Quantitys were small and I hade room enough I have putt up in your Brother Thomas Case makeing noe doubt hee will upon your demand deliver them to you which I thought a better way and lesse Charge then to putt them up by themselves. I have [*blot*: ad]vised and agreed with both your Brothers to trade with them upon another foot as they will informe you and if you choose rather to deale soe will doe the same with you for the future of which pray signifye your mind by the next opertunity. You see have charged nothing for the Empl ad Herniam[1] because you say it was omitted tho I feare you overlooked it in unpacking the Chest for I am pretty confident it was sent. This is the Needfull but hearty Service, etc.   JC

122 MR THOMAS PHYLLIPS, BARBADOS

Sept 6 1717

SIR

Yours of Aprill 9th I have before me and by Advice sent June 12 per Capt Sprigmore to your Brother John I desyred him to advise you that I designed to prepare and forward your Invoyce as soon as possible Could, and upon what Conditions, of which I hope hee aquainted you with. This serves to Inclose Invoyce and Bill of Loading the said goods conteined in your Invoyce, herewith forwarded to you per Capt Combes in the Grocer Friggott which I wish well to your hands and every way to your Content and Satisfaction which I have endeavoured all I can. You'l observe the goods are upon your risque out and home and that there is a double Invoyce of them: one of the

---

1 *Emplastrum ad Herniam*, a plaster of myriad ingredients including galls, pomegranate peels, litharge of gold, dragon's blood, ship pitch, etc. Though intended for hernia, Salmon also recommended it to strengthen joints, prevent abortions and stop fluxes (*Pharmacopoeia* 686-7).

Druggs and Medicines without any advance onely charged as low as we sell them for ready money here to any Chapmen; the other Invoyce Containes those goods out of my way and which I bought as hard as I could with ready money for which have advanced on the first cost onely 12 perCent which I am confident is farr lesse then any one in London would have done. The Conditions you knew are to pay for them here in Sterling money in 9 Months time. If you find it more difficult to get a Bill for that sume you may Ship goods: Sugars, Cotton, or Aloes which you please and I will dispose of them to the best advantage I can and give your Account Credit for the produce and send you the Ballance. I desire you to bee very carefull in opening the case that none of the small parcells bee lost or overlookt among the Hay which may very easyly bee done. I am sure everything is put up accept the Unguentum Decameron Mindereri[1] 2 lbs which I cannott tell what you meane by, I never heard of such a thing nor cannott meet with any one that ever did. In your next you must advice where the receipt is to bee found for there is noe such thing in use here. I have taken all possible care about your Instruments and doubt not they will all prove very good soe as may incourage a farther Correspondance which shall bee willingly settled by me. You will find 5 or 6 things in your Case for your Brother William which please to deliver to him, they are all writt upon. There was roome in your Case for them and soe thought being the parcell small it was scarce worth while to put them up by themselves and bee att the expence of a sett of Bills of Loading for them. This is the needful etc.   JC

[*in margin*: Note: I writt att the same time to Mr Adams pressing him earnestly to Ballance mine and Sister Braggs account.]

1 A salve prepared from ten juices by Raymund M. Minderer (d. 1621), an Augsburg physician famous for his *spiritus mindereri*. *Unguentum decameron* was recommended to cleanse and heal open wounds. The full recipe had been translated in 1674 in Minderer's *Medicina Militaris or a Body of Military Medicines Experimented* (London 1674) 105-6. A second English edition was published in 1687, suggesting that his work was not unknown in London. See also OED, s.v. 'Mindererus'; *Biographisches Lexikon der hervorragenden Ärtze* 4 vols. (Berlin 1929-33) 4: 215.

Appendix

COMPLETE LIST OF THE LETTERS

1 Thomas Barton, Salem, Mass., 3 March 1709/10
2 Samuel Proctor, Antigua, 13 March 1709/10
3 Habijah Savage, Boston, Mass., 3 March 1709/10
4 Conrade Adams, Barbados, 13 March 1709/10
5 Capt. James Pitts, Boston, Mass., 2 March 1709/10
6 Thomas Little, Plymouth, Mass., 9 March 1709/10
7 William Weaver, Barbados, 3 March 1709/10
8 Joseph Ward, Barbados, 13 March 1709/10
9 Habijah Savage, Boston, Mass., 27 June 1710
10 Habijah Savage, Boston, Mass., 1 August 1710
11 Thomas Greaves, Charlestown, Mass., 1 August 1710
12 William Little, Boston, Mass., 1 August 1710
13 Thomas Barton, Salem, Mass., 1 August 1710
14 George Greemes, Barbados, 20 December 1710
15 Conrade Adams, Barbados, 20 December 1710
16 Conrade Adams, Barbados, 22 February 1710/11
17 William Phillips, Barbados, 20 December 1710
18 Richard Eyton, Jamaica, 3 January 1710/11
19 Thomas Perkins, Jamaica, 18 January 1710/11
20 Edward Bulkley, Madras, India, 22 January 1710/11
21 Waterhouse Freenly, Jamaica, 13 February 1710/11
22 Capt. Samuel Vassall, Jamaica, 13 February 1710/11
23 Thomas Barton, Salem, Mass., 3 March 1710/11
24 Thomas Barton, Salem, Mass., 13 April 1711
25 Habijah Savage, Boston, Mass., 3 March 1710/11

26 Habijah Savage, Boston, Mass., 5 April 1711
27 William Little, Boston, Mass., 5 March 1710/11
28 George Jackson, Piscataqua, New Hampshire, 5 March 1710/11
29 George Jackson, Piscataqua, New Hampshire, 18 April 1711
30 Thomas Little, Plymouth, Mass., 5 March 1710/11
31 Conrade Adams, Barbados, 3 April 1712
32 William Phillips, Barbados, 3 April 1712
33 George Greemes, Barbados, 7 April 1712
34 Habijah Savage, Boston, Mass., 4 ? April 1712
35 Habijah Savage, Boston, Mass., 14 May 1712
36 William Little, Boston, Mass., 15 April 1712
37 Thomas Barton, Salem, Mass., 14 May 1712
38 Thomas Little, Plymouth, Mass., 14 May 1712
39 George Jackson, Piscataqua, New Hampshire, 14 May 1712
40 George Jackson, Piscataqua, New Hampshire, 22 July 1712
41 Habijah Savage, Boston, Mass., 24 July 1712
42 Habijah Savage, Boston, Mass., 25 August, 1712
43 Thomas Barton, Salem, Mass., 24 July 1712
44 Thomas Barton, Salem, Mass., 25 August 1712
45 John Emerson, Newcastle, New Hampshire, 25 July 1712
46 William Little, Boston, Mass., 25 August 1712
47 Conrade Adams, Barbados, 27 February 1712/13
48 Dr Frank Jemmett, Barbados, 2 March 1712/13
49 William Phillips, Barbados, 2 March 1712/13
50 Thomas Perkins, Jamaica, 8 April 1713
51 Thomas Barton, Salem, Mass., 9 April 1713
52 Habijah Savage, Boston, Mass., 16 April 1713
53 Thomas Greaves, Charlestown, Mass., 16 April 1713
54 William Little, Boston, Mass., 25 July 1713
55 William Little, Boston, Mass., 3 October 1713
56 Habijah Savage, Boston, Mass., 3 October 1713
57 Thomas Perkins, Jamaica, 12 December 1713
58 Samuel Proctor, Antigua, 8 January 1713/14
59 Dr Robert Anderson, Barbados, 23 January 1713/14
60 Conrade Adams & Co., Barbados, 23 January, 1713/14
61 Habijah Savage, Boston, Mass., 18 February 1713/14
62 Thomas Barton, Salem, Mass., 18 February 1713/14
63 James Henderson, New York, 13 March 1713/14
64 Capt. John Tucker, New York, 13 March 1713/14

65 Thomas Barton, Salem, Mass., 22 April 1714
66 Thomas Greaves, Charlestown, Mass., 22 April 1714
67 George Jackson, Piscataqua, New Hampshire, 22 April 1714
68 Habijah Savage, Boston, Mass., 22 April 1714
69 Habijah Savage, Boston, Mass., 28 July 1714
70 John Nicholls, Boston, Mass., 28 July 1714
71 William Rand, Boston, Mass., 28 July 1714
72 Dr Robert Anderson, Barbados, 24 August 1714
73 Conrade Adams, Barbados, 24 August 1714
74 Habijah Savage, Boston, Mass., 4 December 1714
75 Thomas Greaves, Charlestown, Mass., 15 March 1714/15
76 John Nicholls, Boston, Mass., 17 March 1714/15
77 Conrade Adams, Barbados, 14 March 1714/15
78 William Phillips, Barbados, 15 March 1714/15
79 Thomas Barton, Salem, Mass., March 1714/15
80 William Rand, Boston, Mass., 22 March 1714/15
81 Habijah Savage, Boston, Mass., 18 March 1714/15
82 James Henderson, New York, 6 April 1715
83 Thomas Barton, Salem, Mass., 22 August 1715
84 Habijah Savage, Boston, Mass., 22 August 1715
85 John Nicholls, Boston, Mass., 22 August 1715
86 Thomas Perkins, Jamaica, 25 August 1715
87 Dr Nathaniel Lucas, Barbados, 18 October 1715
88 Dr Frank Jemmett, Barbados, 18 October 1715
89 William Phillips, Barbados, 18 October 1715
90 Conrade Adams & Co., Barbados, 18 October 1715
91 George Stewart, Boston, Mass., 18 February 1715/16
92 Thomas Barton, Salem, Mass., 18 February 1715/16
93 Habijah Savage, Boston, Mass., 18 February 1715/16
94 Thomas Greaves, Charlestown, Mass., 30 April 1716
95 William Rand, Boston, Mass., 30 April 1716
96 Habijah Savage, Boston, Mass., 30 April 1716
97 John Nicholls, Boston, Mass., 30 April 1716
98 William Arbuckle, Jamaica, 16 August 1716
99 Crawford & Poyntz, Jamaica, 18 August 1716
100 Habijah Savage, Boston, Mass., 25 August 1716
101 William Rand, Boston, Mass., 25 August 1716
102 Thomas Greaves, Charlestown, Mass., 25 August 1716
103 Thomas Barton, Salem, Mass., 25 August 1716

104 Habijah Savage, Boston, Mass., 28 September 1716
105 Thomas Greaves, Charlestown, Mass., 28 September 1716
106 William Rand, Boston, Mass., 28 September 1716
107 Thomas Barton, Salem, Mass., 28 September 1716
108 William Phillips Jr., Barbados, 8 November 1716
109 George Stewart, Boston, Mass., 26? February 1716/17
110 John Nicholls, Boston, Mass., 1 March 1716/17
111 Thomas Barton, Salem, Mass., 2 March 1716/17
112 William Little, Boston, Mass., 17 April 1717
113 George Jackson, Piscataqua, New Hampshire, 15 May 1717
114 Thomas Barton, Salem, Mass., 30 May 1717
115 Habijah Savage, Boston, Mass., 3 June 1717
116 John Phillips, Barbados, 12 June 1717
117 John Compton, Boston, Mass., 31 July 1717
118 Habijah Savage, Boston, Mass., 30 July 1717
119 Thomas Barton, Salem, Mass., 31 July 1717
120 John Phillips, Barbados, 6 September 1717
121 William Phillips Jr., Barbados, 6 September 1717
122 Thomas Phillips, Barbados, 6 September 1717

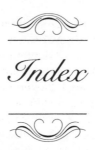

Index

Boldface numbers refer to major descriptions of people and commodities.